I0789787

Why a Book of the Blogs?

When my family doctor told me I probably had a problem and it had to do with my kidneys, maybe Chronic Kidney Disease, my first reaction was to demand in no uncertain terms, "What is it and how did I get it?" Hence, the original title of my blog and the book with which it began.

There are many, many of us out there. By us, I mean those who have Chronic Kidney Disease. Friends and family of CKD patients can gain some insight into the daily travails of living with the disease via this blog, too. I am no expert, but I have read just about every book concerning this problem that I could find. Of course, most medical texts are not included because I couldn't understand them. Most of the kidney disease cookbooks aren't included because I can understand a heavy duty medical text better than I can a cookbook. I even read memoirs and biographies to glean what information I could.

Surprisingly, very few of these books dealt with the early or moderate stages of the disease. These are the stages when we, as patients, are most shocked, confused, depressed and at sea. I didn't want to read about transplants or kidney failure. They scared me and I just wasn't ready to learn about them.

But I did want to know what was happening to me on a daily basis, what the medications that were ordered for me were supposed to do, and what new discoveries there were that might help slow down this deterioration of my kidneys. That's what this blog is about.

The more you know about Chronic Kidney Disease and the more anecdotes you read about other people's relationship with it, the more comfortable you'll feel in the early or moderate stages of having the disease yourself. I wish someone had blogged about it when it was new to me.

I've discovered I have readers all over the world and they're not afraid to tell me what they need to know. I research for them and respond with a blog post, but remind them they need to speak with their nephrologist and/or renal nutritionist before taking any action.

I did write a first book about Chronic Kidney Disease that you'll find referenced many times in the blogs. That book is **What Is It and How Did I Get It? Early Stage Chronic Kidney Disease**. You can find it in print and digital on Amazon.com, as well digital on B & N.com. The first months of the blog and most of the missing blogs are the chapters of the book. Rather than repeat what I'd already written about in the first book, I decided to include only new information in this second book.

I started the blog after a doctor in India contacted me telling me he wanted his patients to have the first book, but sometimes they couldn't even afford the bus fare to the clinic. I suggested I start the blog [Not having a clue how to do that], he translate it, then print it and give it to patients. The idea was that those who could make it to the clinic would bring the printed copies of the blog back to their villages. I wish I had thought to keep that email.

Anyway, that's why the blog was begun on September 3, 2010, but the blogs in this second book begin on February 11, 2011. Once I exhausted the chapters of the book, I didn't want to stop. This is one of the most rewarding services I've ever performed.

You'll notice erratic posting dates until I hit my stride and figured out this needed to be a once a week blog. I've also omitted blog posts which were not in chronological order, but were published in **What Is It and How Did I Get It? Early Stage Chronic Kidney Disease** or were about websites that no longer exist, products that no longer exist, or services that are no longer available. When you see a set of braces rather than quotation marks, it's me inserting my thoughts into an article.

In the interest of keeping the book from becoming mammoth, I've removed the pictures and a great many references to what was happening at that time in my personal life. I also removed my signature closing: "Until next week, keep living your life!" After all, how many times can you read the same sentence in a single book?

When that still didn't shorten the book enough, I removed all notices of past book signings, book talks, Twitter chats, interviews, radio shows, and articles that I'd been involved with. You can't very well go back to the past to attend them, listen to them, or read them from dead links, so why include them I reasoned.

Once I received the proof copy of this book, it was clear that what I had envisioned as one book had to become four. In order to keep reader costs down, the book had to be a paperback. The proof copy was so big that simply opening the book broke the binding.

Enough already! Without further ado, welcome to the first half of the former ***The Book of Blogs: Moderate Stage Chronic Kidney Disease, Part 1*** which is now ***SlowItDownCKD 2011*** and ***SlowItDownCKD 2012.*** To make them even better, each book now has an index thanks to reader feedback. Enjoy your reading.

Keep living your life,
Gail

p.s. Bear, you didn't think I'd forget to thank you for accepting that Monday is reserved for writing the blog, did you? Many thanks for respecting that, you thoughtful husband, you.

Book Review

2/11/11   It's book review day. I'll be reviewing Dr. Tracey I. Marks's *Master Your Sleep: Proven Methods Simplified.* Unfortunately, Dr. Marks hasn't gotten back to me before today to answer my question about how her book specifically applies to early stage Chronic Kidney Disease patients. Ordinarily, that would make me think twice about reviewing her book, but it is possible that she intends to send me that e-mail at a later date. I'm willing to give her the benefit of the doubt.

According to the biography on the back cover of the book Tracey Marks, MD is an Atlanta psychiatrist and psychotherapist who has a special interest in how the mind and body connect to shape our quality of life. Dr. Marks has worked with numerous women struggling to balance their life and work, while also overcoming burnout, depression and other stress-related issues.

Dr. Marks obtained her undergraduate degree from Duke University and her medical degree from the University of Florida. She completed her residency training at The New York Presbyterian Hospital, Cornell Medical Center.

Now that we know who the author is, a discussion of what the book contains is in order. I won't go into too much detail, even though I know I can't spoil a non-fiction by telling too much because this is only a review, not a book report which would tell you a great deal more [Aha! Snuck in a little bit of teaching writing there, didn't I?]

Dr. Marks starts us off with the basics: facts about sleep, what happens if you don't sleep, why you can't sleep [If you can't], and who might need which sleep disorder evaluation. She effortlessly moves into sleep solutions such as medications, and different kinds of therapies: behavioral, cognitive, and bright light. The doctor also includes a chapter on sleep disorders in children and a final, summary chapter to pull together the information in the previous chapters.

She has thoughtfully included many tables, such as sleep needs by age and caffeine concentration in foods tables among others. In addition, Dr. Marks has included copies of both parts of the sleep diary she writes about, the assumption log and the problem-solving worksheet, which are also downloadable from the website mentioned in the appendix.

The book itself is appealing in that it's printed on non-gloss paper and the cover is in muted colors. Most interesting to me was her simple analysis of what was, for the most part, a common sense approach to falling and staying asleep. I had to re-evaluate the common sense part of that sentence when I realized it took me decades to make this material 'common sense' for myself.

As Chronic Kidney Disease patients, we'd be particularly interested in her discussion of how much fluid the bladder holds, how full it needs to be before we feel the urge to urinate, how long different fluids take to pass through our bodies and how to avoid numerous wake-ups to urinate. The following is from that discussion.

Your kidneys will continue to filter your blood overnight but at a much slower rate than during the day.

A really nice touch was the 'Master Your Sleep Cheat Sheet' that is inserted in the book. You don't even have to tear it out. It is stur-dy, portable and quite clear cut.

While I would not necessarily make this book my sleep bible, I did find it helpful. I've already touted some of its wisdom to friends and family who needed the information.

The Doctor Responds and More

2/15/11   Dr. Marks, the author of the book that was reviewed Friday, sent me a response immediately. I laughingly wondered if it truly were sent the second my post was published. While Dr. Marks sent it as a comment, I'm going to actually copy it here.

Hi, thanks for your review. Also, thanks for giving me the benefit of the doubt. As it turns out, I didn't get your question, but I'd be happy to address that now.

Even for people with medical disorders that interfere with sleep, maintaining good sleep hygiene as discussed in chapter 6 is important. I like your comment about common sense information. I tend to err on the side of assuming people know the things I know because it's become so routine for me. Then when I see a new patient who is doing lots of stuff to sabotage their sleep, I'm reminded that these tips may be intuitive, but that doesn't always translate to common practice.

So attending to sleep hygiene – all aspects of it as best you can, specifically helps the chronic kidney sufferer.

Next, if a person progresses to have other medical complications such as chronic fatigue, pain or depression, the sufferer should consider sleeping medication. Chapter 5 discusses the different medication options and this information can help you make an informed choice when you talk to your doctor.

As you know, people on dialysis can develop insomnia due to sleep apnea. I only discuss sleep apnea briefly in the book. The book is really designed to be a self-help tool. Since sleep apnea requires professional help, I did not elaborate much except to give information on the symptoms, the sleep study that diagnoses it and treatment options.

Lastly, although I'm a proponent of not taking medications when you don't need to (even though I'm a medical doctor), I believe those with chronic medical conditions are just the population of people who need sleeping medication long term.

That said – medications don't always work all the time. Many of them lose their effectiveness. So anything you can do behaviorally to help your sleep is advantageous. All this to say, I also think the section on sleep restriction would be helpful to the person with Chronic Kidney Disease who has broken sleep all through the night DESPITE being on sleep medication.

One more thing, people with kidney disease can end up with day-night reversal where they are up all night and sleeping during the day. This can really get in the way of doctors' appointments, dialysis if applicable, and other life commitments. This is where light therapy that I discuss in Chapter 8 may be extremely helpful.

Bright light has a powerful effect on the body clock and helping people sleep at the right times. More recent research that post-dates the book supports the use of light boxes also for non-seasonal depression. This is exciting to me because it's possible the light therapy can not only help regulate one's sleep but lift the depression that kidney disease sufferers can develop. Okay, I think that's it. Thanks for the question!

And thanks to Dr. Marks for her quick response once she did receive the question.

Not Again!

2/18/11 In one of those little flukes during which I didn't receive my nephrologist's report until a few weeks after the doctor visit and didn't catch everything he said during the visit, I noticed a colonoscopy was recommended. But I had one only eight years ago! When I called the nephrologist's office to speak to his M.A. [Medical Assist-ant] in an effort to find out why I needed this test, it was explained to me that the fatigue I'd been experiencing just might be from polyps.

That didn't sound right to me so I dutifully made an appointment with the gastroenterologist, and while there, had a long, involved discussion with him. He wisely allowed me to do most of the talking to see if he could get a handle on the nephrologist's reason for wanting this test performed, but couldn't.

Was it my failure to understand the M.A.? Could be, but just to be certain AND to find out which drugs I would be allowed since I now have CKD and was going to be 'put out' – oh, Lord, I hope that's nothing akin to being 'put down' – for the experience , this specialist agreed to call the other specialist.

Here it is almost two weeks later and I've heard nothing from either of them. Apparently, my nephrologist is on vacation and we're waiting for his return. So, of course, I started research-ing on my own. I still can't quite figure out why I'm having the test since I couldn't find anything about polyps contributing to fatigue in CKD patients [Which doesn't mean the information isn't there – it may have been too technical for me to understand], but I did discover the following warning on the National Kidney Foundation's site.

Oral Sodium Phosphate Safety Alerts

Patients with Chronic Kidney Disease (CKD) who use bowel cleansing products should be aware of a recent warning issued by the FDA for a type of sudden loss of kidney function or acute kidney injury, as well as, blood mineral disturbances. Phosphate crystal deposition in the kidneys causes the loss of kidney function, which can lead to kidney failure. The medical term for this condition is acute phosphate nephropathy.

The warning relates to the use of bowel cleansing agents, called sodium phosphate (OSP) products as laxatives or in preparation for colonoscopy. OSPs are available both with and without a prescription and are taken by mouth. These products can cause phosphate nephropathy. Oral sodium phosphates clear the bowel by making bowel movements frequent, loose and runny. These agents work by causing fluid loss so it is recommended to patients that they drink large quantities of clear liquids as part of the bowel preparation. Symptoms of acute phosphate nephropathy are:

- Lethargy
- Drowsiness
- Decreased urination
- Swelling of ankles, feet and legs

Early on, people may not have any symptoms at all. Anyone at high risk for this condition should have their kidney function monitored by their doctor. Visicol® and OsmoPrep® are available by prescription only. Other similar OSP products are non-prescription, and can be used as a laxative at low doses.

Children under 18 years should not use these products alone or in combination with other laxatives containing sodium phosphate. Other groups who are at risk for acute phosphate nephropathy are:

- People over 55
- CKD patients
- People who are dehydrated
- People who have bowel obstruction, delayed bowel emptying
- or active colitis
- People taking medications such as diuretics, angiotensin converting enzyme [ACE] inhibitors, angiotensin receptor blockers [ARBs], and inflammation and pain relief medications such as nonsteroidal anti-inflammatory drugs [NSAIDs])

The FDA requested that the manufacturer of Visicol® and Osmo-Prep®, Salix Pharmaceuticals

- Add a black boxed warning to the pharmacy package insert for these products
- Develop and distribute a medication guide for patients that is easier for most patients to understand than package inserts
- Arrange a post-marketing trial to assess the risks to patients taking OSP products

Non-prescription OSP products have a long history of safety when used as laxatives and will still be available over the counter. *However, because of the recent warning by the FDA, those OSP products should only be used as laxatives and not for bowel cleansing. The FDA suggests consumers should get a prescription from a health care professional when thinking about having a bowel cleansing.*

The U.S. Preventive Services Task Force (USPSTF) strongly recommends that clinicians screen men and women 50 years of age or older for colorectal cancer with one of several tests, including colonoscopy. If your doctor recommends colonoscopy, concerns about bowel cleansing should not prevent you from undergoing colon cancer screening. Colon cancer is treatable when the disease is caught early and the best treatment is to identify and remove precancerous polyps before they progress to cancer.

A high-quality and safe colon cleansing preparation is important for colon cancer screening using colonoscopy. There are other FDA-approved alternatives to OSP for bowel preparation prior to colonoscopy that may be safer for some patients, but may not always clean the bowel adequately. Patients should discuss the risks of the preparation and procedure, versus the benefits of the screening to determine the best bowel cleaning agent for their age, and risk conditions noted above.

More than 26 million American adults and thousands of American children have Chronic Kidney Disease. Most do not know they have this condition.
Date Reviewed: July 2009

July, 2009, was 18 months ago yet I've found no updates anywhere on the internet. Whether or not I'm satisfied with what my nephrologist tells the gastroenterologist or what the gastroenterologist tells me, I intend to bring this information with me to the gastroenterologist BEFORE the procedure and certainly bring it to the attention of the nephrologist. After all, I am responsible for managing my own health issues.

Medhelp's Advice

2/25/11   Information seems to jump onto my screen when I'm not even looking for it. For example, Medhelp.org periodically sends me e-mails. Recently, I wasn't happy with still having high blood pressure after all these years even though it's controlled. Bang! Medhelp sent me an e-mail about the worst and best foods to eat when you have high blood pressure.

While most of this information is already in my renal diet arsenal, there were a few items I didn't know about since I was following the renal diet, not one for high blood pressure. Just goes to show that you learn something new every day.

As to Medhelp's advice: among the drinks to avoid are soft drinks – even low-calorie ones, iced tea, and fruit punch. I stick to filtered water and coffee so it made no difference to me, but you might be drinking these.

From following the renal diet, we already know to avoid packaged and processed meat products, bacon, sausage, bologna and hot dogs. Doing so will also help prevent your high blood pressure from rising further. I ate a hot dog just the other day [Basically I just gave in to that old devil peer pressure.] and was both surprised and delighted that I no longer had a taste for them. Just as with the renal diet, your tastes will change as you get used to eating only the foods on your specific diet.

For those who drink, binge drinking can raise your blood pressure. That one was news to me, but I decided it made sense. You have to decide for yourself. I don't drink, so this is like judging new places as an armchair traveler.

Refrigerated biscuits and crescent rolls made the no-no list too since they contain trans-fat which is 'associated with the risk of high blood pressure in middle-aged and older women.' In general, foods containing hydrogenated oil in the ingredients list should be avoided since that indicates they contain some trans-fat, even if it's not listed on the label.

There is a controversy as to whether or not coffee raises blood pressure. I, for one, am not giving up my 16 ounces of caffeine a day until this is proven. I'm careful about my eating, but I'm human! I love my coffee.

I don't know if it's possible to get or make a low sodium pizza, but pizza as we know it can really raise your blood pressure due to the excessive amounts of sodium in it.

What foods are good for hindering high blood pressure? Fruits and vegetables since they're packed with potassium but be careful. You know as Chronic Kidney Disease patients you need to watch those potassium levels. And continue to avoid star fruit which can be toxic to us.

Also using herbs and spices instead of salt, another tactic we already employ since we have CKD. Again, be careful about which ones you choose. You don't want to hinder high blood pressure at the cost of more kidney damage.

Stick to low-fat dairy products, not that we have a lot of choice in dairy products as CKD patients, to aid in hindering high blood pressure.

I've got to admit I found myself overwhelmed when I first received the renal diet three years ago, but eventually got the hang of it. In January, I was given the latest update of that diet and am still trying to incorporate the changes into my diet. I'm back to a lot of looking foods up on the list to see if they are now permissible or if they were the permissible ones which are now considered harmful to CKD patients.

When I looked at Medhelp's suggestions to avoid increasing the high blood pressure I already have and some food suggestions for hindering high blood pressure, I was pleased to discover they only necessitated one or two changes to my already challenging dietary restrictions.

Take a good look at the suggestions. Maybe there are one or two that will come easily to you. Then take a look at the ones "You know it don't come easy." [Thank you, Ringo Starr, for the right words at the right time.] and give them a try one at a time.

Dear Abby Speaks

3/8/11   Thursday is World Kidney Day, while March in National Kidney Month. There's a reason there's such attention being paid to our kidneys. *The Arizona Republic* carried a 'Dear Abby' column about kidney disease. With thanks to Amy Vlasity for bringing it to my attention and Dear Abby, that column is today's blog.

Dear Abby: Like many other young adults, I was too busy establishing a career during my 20s and early 30s to care much about diet and exercise.

I felt healthy, so I saw no need to change my lifestyle. My doctor had told me my blood pressure was elevated during a number of my yearly physical exams, but I didn't ask any questions and took no action. Then one morning, I walked into my doctor's office complaining of a severe headache and nausea. I was sent to the hospital with a dangerously high blood pressure reading. After just a few tests, I was told I had Chronic Kidney Disease.

Even though it can be silent and cause no symptoms, high blood pressure should not be ignored. It is a leading cause of kidney disease, and because I didn't pay attention, my kidneys began to shut down. Abby, please tell your readers who are at risk for Chronic Kidney Disease (and that's anyone with high blood pressure, diabetes or a family history of CKD) to check how their kidneys are functioning. I found out – too
late – how important it is.

- Aziza M., New York City

Dear Aziza: Of course I will pass on your warning. According to the National Kidney Foundation, more than 26 million adults and thousands of American children have Chronic Kidney Disease – and most of them don't know they have it. In addition, millions of people who have diabetes, hypertension and other diseases are unaware that they too are at risk for developing it.

Thursday is World Kidney Day. The National Kidney Foundation is offering free screenings during the month of March through the Kidney Early Evaluation Program in cities and towns around the country.

With more than 50 local offices nationwide, the NKF provides early-detection screenings and other vital patient and community services. I went to their website and found what looked like a comprehensive list of screening areas throughout the country, but didn't see my home state. That's when I noticed the area directly above the list where you can enter your zip code, hit submit and a drop down list of local centers will appear.

Today's blog will stay short and sweet so you get the message: urge everyone you know to get themselves checked. There are no symptoms until you have lost MOST of your kidney function. Don't wait, please.

Nima's Side of The Equation

3/11/11   You've probably read my mentioning that my older daughter is also a writer. Nima had an intriguing idea: in honor of National Kidney Month, she wanted to write a guest blog about being someone who loves someone else with Chronic Kidney Disease. I was touched by the thought.

The Other Side of the CKD Equation
By Nima Beckie (*Also known as the daughter of Gail Rae*)

In honor of National Kidney Month, I asked my mother if she would let me write a guest blog on what it's like to be on the other side of The CKD equation, and where family members and loved ones of people living with CKD could find resources aimed for them. And now, without further ado, I bring you my side of the equation.

I have to admit when my mother first told me she had CKD I freaked out ever so slightly. My knowledge of CKD was minimal, if that and it took more than a few times of Ma telling me that CKD was in fact manageable and not a death sentence to calm down.

After I'd wrapped my brain around that, I started doing my own research about what exactly CKD was, and how I could be supportive as a family member.

I knew of the walks that took place nationally to raise money for Kidney Awareness since a friend had started organizing a team locally for an annual New York walk. That started to spark my interest in regard to other ways I could be supportive of CKD awareness. I soon learned that green was the color of the Kidney Awareness ribbon. While I've seen many various Kidney Ribbon items sold (i.e. jewelry, magnets, mugs, pencils, etc.), I've yet to find a real ribbon that wasn't sold in bulk.

One thing I had to get used to was reminding myself to mention at doctor visits that a parent has CKD, and to please take blood work to keep an eye on my own GFR levels. Every now and then I'd also get a helpful reminder from Ma right before a doctor visit.

I then started to look for resources for families of CKD patients. I found quite a few groups for those living with CKD and their family members, but, only a few just for family members. I still would encourage you to take a look at both Yahoo Groups and Google Groups for support forums. Quite a lot of the information that I did find came from a bunch of the websites that are listed on this blog.

I also have another resource that not everyone else has: I have a mother who is also writing a very detailed book about her experiences with discovering she had CKD. Getting a chance to read the manuscript of her upcoming book was probably where I got the meat and potatoes of my CKD education.

So, in the end, my education of CKD went from minimal to far beyond what you'd learn in a high school, or even in some cases, college biology class. For those out there that have a loved one that was recently diagnosed with CKD, I'm not going to tell you not to freak out, but I am going to tell you to educate yourself about CKD. Believe me, you'll freak out far less.

Also, don't be afraid to ask questions about what you can do to help and what you should know about how CKD affects your family member or loved one. I was always worried about tiring my mother out until she finally explained to me that as long as she gets a chance to lay down/nap before we go out, she's usually fine.

I'm blessed I have a great mother who's been there for me through thick and thin, now I have a chance to be there for her. (Now you know one of the reasons I'm so proud of my daughter.)

What Did You Say?

3/15/11   In honor of National Kidney Month [Not to be confused with World Kidney Day], I searched the web to see what new information I could find. When I did find it, you could have heard a pin drop – or maybe not. Now I understand why my children have been begging me to get my hearing tested.

The following appeared on Yahoo's PRWEB on Monday, March 14, 2011. I took the online test mentioned in the article and, sure enough, I need to see an audiologist. Consider taking the online test yourself after you read this not very well known information about CKD patients.

People with Chronic Kidney Disease Should Have Their Hearing Checked:
March is National Kidney Month

People with Chronic Kidney Disease (CKD) should take the Across America Hearing Check Challenge—a free, quick, and confidential online hearing test at http://www.hearingcheck.org. The non-profit Better Hearing Institute (BHI) is offering the test as part of its effort to raise awareness of the link between Chronic Kidney Disease and hearing loss. March is National Kidney Month. BHI's online test will help people determine if they need a comprehensive hearing check by a hearing professional.

Research shows that hearing loss is common in people with moderate Chronic Kidney Disease. As published in the American Journal of Kidney Diseases and highlighted on the National Kidney Foundation web site, a team of Australian researchers found that older adults with moderate Chronic Kidney Disease (CKD) have a higher prevalence of hearing loss than those of the same age without CKD.

According to the National Kidney Foundation, an Australian research team assessed more than 2,900 individuals aged 50 and older, including 513 with moderate Chronic Kidney Disease. Of those with CKD, more than 54 percent reported some level of hearing loss compared to only 28 percent of the rest of the group. Nearly 30 percent of the CKD participants showed severe hearing loss compared with only 10 percent of the non-CKD participants.

"Unaddressed hearing loss can have very significant consequences on a person's life and greatly undermine quality of life," said Sergei Kochkin, PhD, BHI's executive director. "We need to alert people with Chronic Kidney Disease of their potential for hearing loss as a result of their disease and encourage hearing screenings as part of their routine medical care to help optimize their quality of life."

Also according to the National Kidney Foundation, 26 million American adults have CKD and millions of others are at increased risk. But early detection can help prevent the progression of kidney disease to kidney failure.

Referencing the Australian study, Dr. Kerry Willis, Senior Vice President of Scientific Activities at the National Kidney Foundation stated: "These findings could lead to a modification of the usual care of people with CKD. Earlier clinical hearing assessments and fitting of hearing aids in CKD patients can improve quality of life and lead to better management of underlying conditions which could, in turn, potentially preserve hearing function."

About Hearing Loss
Approximately one in 10 Americans, or 34 million people, have some degree of hearing loss. Yet, fewer than 15 percent of physicians today ask patients if they have any hearing problems.

Numerous studies have linked untreated hearing loss to a wide range of physical and emotional conditions, including impaired memory and ability to learn new tasks, reduced alertness, increased risk to personal safety, irritability, negativism, anger, fatigue, tension, stress, depression, and diminished psychological and overall health.

Fortunately, the vast majority of people with hearing loss can be helped with hearing aids. And nine out of ten hearing aid users report improvements in their quality of life.

Founded in 1973, BHI conducts research and engages in hearing health education with the goal of helping people with hearing loss benefit from proper treatment.

It's Still National Kidney Month

3/19/11   In honor of National Kidney Month, I've been trying to find current articles with new information or information that's important to hear over and over again. Today, The National Kidney Organization provided the following article.

Despite a Diagnosis, Many Kidney Disease Patients Remain Unaware

March 1, 2011—Many people diagnosed with Chronic Kidney Disease do not know they have the disease, according to a new report published in the March issue of the *American Journal of Kidney Diseases*, the official Journal of the National Kidney Foundation.

Researchers at Vanderbilt University Medical Center in Nashville, Tennessee, surveyed 401 people with kidney disease attending a nephrology clinic. More than 75% of participants had stage 3 Chronic Kidney Disease or above. While 94% of patients surveyed were aware they had a kidney "problem," more than 30% were unaware they had a serious, potentially life–threatening disease. All of the patients surveyed were under the care of a kidney specialist, or nephrologist.

"The lack of awareness of Chronic Kidney Disease among those who are affected appears to be greater than other health conditions," said study co–author Dr. Julie Anne Wright from Vanderbilt's Division of Nephrology and Hypertension. "Even when patients are under the care of specialists, they frequently have a limited understanding of fundamental topics, including symptoms, the course of kidney disease and risk factors such as diabetes and hypertension. This study highlights the need for providers to ensure that communication is not only delivered but understood between all parties involved."

Beyond diagnosis awareness, results of the 34–question survey also showed that 78% of participants did not know that the disease may progress with no symptoms. More than 34% were unaware that they were at increased risk for heart disease and 32% did not know that the kidneys make urine.

"Because kidney disease may be silent, it's critically important that anyone at risk—those with high blood pressure, diabetes or a family history of kidney disease—get their kidney function checked regularly. This report shows that most people are not aware that kidney disease often has no symptoms, both in the early stages and even in the more advanced stages. Yet there are steps people can take to save their health if they are aware that they're at risk or that they have Chronic Kidney Disease," says Joseph Vassalotti, MD, National Kidney Foundation's Chief Medical Officer.

Nearly all therapies aimed at preventing kidney disease progression and decreasing associated complications rely heavily on patient self–care. "Once diagnosed, people can take action to prevent the disease from getting worse," continued Vassalotti. "Partnering with the clinician for risk factor control of diabetes and high blood pressure, as well as avoidance of medications that are toxic to the kidneys, can help slow the progression of the disease." March is National Kidney Month, March 10 is World Kidney Day and the National Kidney Foundation will be offering free screenings for those at risk around the country through its Kidney Early Evaluation Program (KEEP). The National Kidney Foundation is dedicated to preventing and treating kidney and urinary tract diseases, improving the health and well-being of individuals and families affected by these diseases and increasing availability of all organs for transplantation.

It's me again. Did you catch that these people did not know they have Chronic Kidney Disease? That's why you MUST get copies of your lab reports and doctor visit reports and learn to read them. Ask your doctor the questions reading these reports raises.

Remember Smokey the Bear says that only you can prevent forest fires? Guess what. Only you can prevent your Chronic Kidney Disease from rapidly getting worse. It's your life; be responsible for it.

Kidney Month Redux

3/22/11   Still in keeping with the spirit of National Kidney Month, I'm posting the National Kidney Disease Education Program's (NKDEP) suggestions. NKDEP is an initiative of the National Institute of Diabetes and Digestive and Kidney Diseases (NIDDK), National Institutes of Health (NIH), U.S. Department of Health & Human Services (DHHS).

10 things you can do to protect your kidneys and help family and friends protect theirs.

If you have diabetes, high blood pressure, or a family history of kidney failure, get your blood and urine checked for kidney disease.

At your next family gathering, talk to loved ones with diabetes and high blood pressure about getting tested for kidney disease.

Learn how to keep your kidneys healthy.

Educate your faith-based community about the kidney connection.

Use spices, herbs and sodium-free seasonings in place of salt.

For those recently diagnosed with kidney disease, find out about the basics of kidney disease and what it means for you.

Watch videos to hear about the different treatment options for kidney failure.

Health care professionals: Learn more about two key markers for Chronic Kidney Disease: urine albumin and estimated glomerular filtration rate.

Become an organ donor.

Enjoy the researching.

National Kidney Month Continues

3/25/11   Continuing the celebration of National Kidney Month, today we visit DaVita. Notice: only the information pertinent to Early Stage Chronic Kidney Disease is included in today's blog.

March is National Kidney Month…. DaVita has teamed with The Kidney TRUST, an organization that aims to benefit the estimated 31 million adults living in the United States who have Chronic Kidney Disease (CKD), as well as the 550,000 Americans with end stage renal disease (ESRD) who need dialysis or a kidney transplant, to help raise awareness about kidney disease.

Chronic Kidney Disease develops when kidneys lose their ability to remove waste and maintain fluid and chemical balances in the body. The severity of Chronic Kidney Disease depends on how well the kidneys filter wastes from the blood. It can progress quickly or take many years to develop.

More than 31 million adults in the US – **ONE IN SIX** [My capitalization and bolding.] – have Chronic Kidney Disease and most of them are not even aware of it. Often there are no symptoms until kidney disease reaches the later stages, including kidney failure.

Risk factors for Chronic Kidney Disease

High-risk populations include those with diabetes, high blood pressure, cardiovascular disease and family history of kidney disease. Eleven percent of the U.S. population has diabetes, the number one cause of kidney disease. One out of three Americans has high blood pressure, the second leading cause of kidney disease.

More than 32 percent of kidney failure patients are African American. Other high-risk groups include Hispanics, Pacific Islanders, Native Americans and seniors 65 and older.

Who should be screened for Chronic Kidney Disease?

Anyone 18 years old or older with diabetes, high blood pressure, cardiovascular disease or a family history of kidney disease should be screened for kidney disease. If you live in an area that is offering a free screening, plan to attend. If not, visit your doctor and ask that you be screened for Chronic Kidney Disease.

What is involved in a kidney screening?

Because there are often no symptoms of kidney disease, laboratory tests are critical. When you get a screening, a trained technician will draw blood that will be tested for creatinine, a waste product. If kidney function is abnormal, creatinine levels will increase in the blood, due to decreased excretion of creatinine in the urine. Your glomerular filtration rate (GFR) will then be calculated, which factors in age, gender, creatinine and ethnicity. The GFR indicates the person's stage of Chronic Kidney Disease which provides an evaluation of kidney function.

Treatment for Chronic Kidney Disease

In many cases, kidney failure can be prevented or delayed through early detection and proper treatment of underlying diseases, such as diabetes and high blood pressure to slow additional damage to the kidneys. Also helpful are an eating plan with the right amounts of sodium, fluid and protein. Additionally, one should exercise and avoid dehydration. Treating diabetes and high blood pressure will slow additional damage to kidneys.

The Last Blog for National Kidney Month

3/29/11   The Kidney TRUST was mentioned in one of the previous National Kidney Month blogs. I had quickly checked it out to make certain it was legit before I included it in that blog and then decided to research it more thoroughly. I liked what I read.

According to its website:

The Kidney TRUST aims to benefit the 31 million American adults living with Chronic Kidney Disease (CKD), as well as the 506,000 Americans with kidney failure that require dialysis or a kidney transplant. The TRUST was formed to increase awareness of kidney disease through public education and testing programs so that progression of CKD to kidney failure can be delayed or prevented.

The Kidney TRUST was founded in 2006 by DaVita Inc., a leading provider of kidney care in the United States. The Kidney TRUST is an independent, nonprofit organization that believes everyone should be empowered to take a proactive role in their health. Toward that end, the TRUST is seeking to reduce the progression of Chronic Kidney Disease (CKD) through free, rapid screening in non-medical settings and to provide financial assistance to people affected by CKD.

The goal of the TRUST's free rapid-testing program, which was launched in October 2007, is to identify individuals who have signs of kidney impairment. Along with learning their screening results onsite, participants receive materials that offer education about CKD and its prevention and are encouraged to seek medical follow-up as appropriate. The TRUST's screening program is carried out in non-medical settings such as large employer workplaces and community health fairs.

Giving In Order To Take?

4/8/11 I've mentioned before that I live in Arizona. I've mentioned before that our governor, Janet Brewer, has decided that organ transplants are elective surgery for AHCCCS [Arizona Health Care Cost Containment System] members. This is the state's Medicaid program.

Now it seems she's changed her mind... at a price, that is. According to our local paper, The Arizona Republic, in a front page article on Thursday, March 31, 2011,

...Brewer also wants lawmakers to restore funding for certain organ transplants.

These are the same organ transplants she eliminated coverage for last fall and for that she's come under severe criticism – especially after several well publicized deaths resulted from the lack of a transplant.

While that may sound like good news, the title of this front page article is **Ariz. asking feds to OK cuts**

"What cuts?" you may ask. "Oh, it's only cuts for lower-income people – nothing that concerns you and me." I've heard people say just that. I think they may be forgetting that people are people no matter what their income level is.

And what are these cuts? According to the article by Mary K. Reinhart and Ginger Rough, they are as follows.

- Freezing enrollment for childless adults....
- Eliminating the medical expense deduction program....
- Cutting reimbursement rates for hospitals, doctors

and other healthcare providers by 5 percent.... [That's in addition to the 5 percent cut that was due to take effect last Friday.]

- New limits on benefits....
- Mandatory co-payments for parents and children, fees for missed appointments,
- $50 fees for patients who smoke, are obese and fail to follow a plan for managing a chronic disease
- Eliminating state emergency-services funding for people without proof of citizenship....
- Requiring patients to re-enroll every six months instead of annually.

I am not by nature a political person and I'm not even sure I understand all this, so I've been very careful to quote the excerpts from the article I've copied in this blog.

This would reflect a savings of over $362,000 annually, but what about the people who need this help. It never occurred to me when I gave blood to even think about the color of the skin of the person who would be receiving that blood, much less to think about their income level. Wouldn't the same hold true for a kidney [or any other] transplant?

The first sentence of the article is:

Gov. Jan Brewer will formally ask federal health officials today to eliminate more than 160,000 people from the Medicaid rolls under a sweeping plan that would freeze two programs for adults, eliminate coverage for catastrophic care, and impose a range of fees, and limits health-care services for Arizona's indigent.

Wow! We have more "indigent" throughout the country due to the economic times. Can we really deny them transplants [those Brewer doesn't restore.] and healthcare because they were downsized? What about their children?

As a humanitarian rather than a politician trying desperately to balance the state's budget, I do not understand any of this. Of course I agree that those on the welfare rolls need to be on a work program, but that doesn't mean I don't want them to have their health issues attended to. What is our world coming to if we can't take care of each other – especially when it comes to health matters?

Breakthroughs!

4/12/11   One of the members of ***The Transplant Community Outreach*** on Facebook brought this to my attention. He's one of the many people who popped up out of nowhere to offer help when he discovered I was writing a book on early stage Chronic Kidney Disease. The information read:

Medical Breakthrough With A Tiny Device

It could change the way doctors treat diabetes, kidney problems and more. Dr. McGeorge shows you why a tiny device is attracting worldwide attention!

… a stem cell soaked device [If I understood correctly] which will be available in about ten years. The beauty of it is that this device can provide your body with some of the services your diseased kidneys would have.

As soon as I finished viewing the accompanying video, I found the following Info posted from Bioscholar.com by Rex & Linda Maus, the administrators of Facebook's ***The Transplant Community Outreach***. By the way, I write 'Kidney Matters,' for them.

Scottish scientists grow kidneys in lab

Scottish scientists have made a breakthrough in organ transplantation by successfully growing kidneys in a laboratory.

The development could help tackle the tragic shortage of organs for transplant, reports the Scotsman.

Researchers at the University of Edinburgh created the organs by manipulating stem cells – early cells that are the building blocks of the body – to form the structure of a kidney.

They then managed to create kidneys that measure just half a centimetre in length – the same size as a kidney in a foetus, which they hope will be able to grow to maturity after being transplanted into patients' bodies.

The kidneys were grown in the laboratory using a combination of cells from amniotic fluid – the fluid that surrounds all babies in the womb – and animal foetal cells.

The technique holds out the prospect of scientists being able to collect amniotic fluid at birth to be stored until needed at a later date if a patient develops kidney disease.

The patient's own amniotic fluid cells can then be used as the base for creating a new kidney.

Using the patient's own cells will, in theory, also end the problem of rejection that arises when an organ from a deceased donor is used.
The Edinburgh researchers are at the forefront of a global attempt to use stem cells culled from amniotic fluid to create new human kidneys.

Speaking for myself, I'm seriously hopeful after reading about these breakthroughs!

In the Interests of Being Fair….

4/26/11 Previously in this blog, I'd written about the unimaginable cuts made to Arizona's Medicaid program by Arizona's governor, Jan Brewer. I'm no fan of hers, BUT I do believe in being fair. Therefore, I'm posting this article from today's *The Arizona Republic*.

Brewer works to restore transplant coverage

Gov. Jan Brewer's office is open to restoring medical transplant coverage for low-income patients, possibly as part of her effort to overhaul the state's Medicaid program.

Brewer first hinted at the possibility during a trip to Prescott Valley last week.

"There is a possibility that that issue can be addressed," Brewer told *The Republic*. "I would hope that there could be a solution, an agreeable solution. That doesn't mean that's going to happen, but we're working to find a solution."

But it's not clear what kind of support there is for the plan among legislators.

Any plan to restore funding would require Legislative approval, Brewer spokesman Matthew Benson said.

Funding for transplants was not included in the $8.1 billion budget proposal approved by the Arizona Senate earlier this month, but the House has yet to take up the issue and it is generally believed it wants to have an agreement with the Governor's Office before beginning its deliberations.

The transplant money was cut last spring when state lawmakers approved a fiscal 2011 budget that cut funding for optional services provided by the Arizona Health Care Cost Containment System, the state's Medicaid program.

Those cuts, designed to help close a massive budget gap, included coverage of certain transplant surgeries, including bone marrow, kidney, liver problems due to hepatitis C and others. Eliminating the transplant funding saved the state about $1.2 million.

The cuts took effect Oct. 1, and drew unflattering national media attention after Goodyear father Mark Price, a leukemia patient was denied coverage for a bone-marrow transplant. An anonymous donor came forward to pay for the procedure, but Price died Nov. 28 of complications to his disease.

National media reports referenced Arizona and its "death panels." Democratic lawmakers have kept the issue at the forefront this Legislative session, but proposals to reinstate funding have gained little traction.

If Brewer's office can successfully negotiate a deal to reinstate transplant funding, it would mark a stunning reversal of position on the issue. She has repeatedly said there is no money for such procedures given the state's ongoing budget crisis. The governor's Medicaid waiver request is due to be submitted to the Health and Human Service Secretary Kathleen Sebelius this week. Brewer's $500 million proposal would eliminate fewer people from the state's Medicaid rolls by freezing enrollment, requiring patients who remain to pay more for their care and reducing the amount paid to health-care providers.

Monica Coury, an assistant director for AHCCCS, said she could shed little light about the possibility of reinstating transplant funding as part of the Medicaid waiver request, saying that "would have to be the governor's decision." Coury said her office is currently working on the Medicaid waiver proposal and "it doesn't have transplants in it."

Am I assured the transplant money will be restored? No, not yet. Am I hopeful? In a word: very. I'm hoping I'm not once again being a Pollyanna, but I'm also hoping that I'm not the only one concerned about this issue.

Think about it. Unfortunately, if the unthinkable can happen here, who's to say it can't happen in your state, too?

Mozart, Too?

4/29/11   While surfing the web to determine if there were any new developments in the treatment of Chronic Kidney Disease, I found some old news today – old news that struck a chord with me [Pun absolutely intended]. I was on a website that sells genetic decoding, which is in itself an intriguing idea. I did notice a line on the site that mentioned they were not approved by the FDA, but were a private lab. I know nothing more about them except that this bit was included on their site.

Did Mozart die of Kidney Disease?

The famous Austrian composer, Wolfgang Amadeus Mozart (born in 1756), had a short but prolific career before he died on December 5th, 1791, only 35 years old. The circumstances of his death have long been a matter of speculation among musical historians and medical scientists alike. Theories on the cause of his premature death range from infections and head trauma to poisoning and even murder.

According to various reliable sources, Mozart fell seriously ill in September of the year of his death. In spite of his illness, he was initially able to continue working, and conducted the premiere of his famous Opera, The Magic Flute (Die Zauberflöte), in Vienna on September 30th, 1791. His illness gradually intensified and in late November Mozart became bedridden, suffering from severe symptoms such as swelling, pain, and vomiting, seen in the advanced stages of Chronic Kidney Disease. Mozart died in Vienna on December 5th, 1791.

According to an article by Dr. E.N. Guillery, published in the *Journal of the American Society of Nephrology* in 1992, kidney failure is indeed one of many theories of Mozart´s terminal illness. In a letter by Mozart´s sister-in-law, who was present during the illness leading to his death, she described that Mozart was unable to turn in bed on account of his swollen condition and that he described having "already the taste of death" on his tongue. This, according to Dr. Guillery, may have been the foul taste of uremia, or the buildup of waste in the blood due to kidney failure. Dr. Guillery's conclusion however, is that unless further information comes to light, the cause of Mozart's death will remain a mystery.

I researched Dr. Guillery's [a pediatric nephrologist] article and, while I'm not certain I understood all of it since it was so technical, decided the conclusion could be easily under-stood by those of us who are not doctors or scientists.

CONCLUSIONS

There are very few conclusions that can be drawn from this debate. It seems quite possible that Mozart died in renal failure, the "taste of death" he complained of may have been the foul taste of uremia. The presence of edema suggests nephrotic syndrome which makes a glomerulopathy likely or volume overload from renal insufficiency. Karhausen's [e.g. from his article "LR: Mozart in person." Times Liter Suppl 1990; Dec: 21-27, 2 1] inclination to propose a relatively common renal disorder associated with Mozart's well-described ear anomaly seems reasonable. Vesicoureteral reflux [e.g. the abnormal flow of urine from the bladder back into the ureters, usually diagnosed in childhood or infancy] in association with a urinary tract anomaly could have caused nephrotic syndrome. Rheumatic fever and SBE [e.g. subacute bacterial endocarditis] cannot be ruled out and are favored by some. We cannot know what killed Mozart unless significant new information comes to light which is unlikely. One should be gratified that Mozart's music lives on.

I'm not sure if I'm honored to possibly share my disease with Mozart or distressed that he suffered without the help we have today. I'll keep pondering that.

Something Good and Fishy Is Happening Here

5/3/11 Since one of my kidney world contacts brought my attention to Bioscholar.com, I've been going to the site periodically to find interesting, innovative, and imperative news about kidneys. I think I found a winner this time.

New findings offer hope to patients with damaged kidneys
Wednesday, February 2nd, 2011

Scientists have discovered a cell in zebra fish that can be transplanted from one fish to another to regenerate nephrons and improve kidney function.

Many non-mammalian vertebrates generate nephrons throughout their lives and can generate new nephrons following renal injury. Under-standing how non-mammalian vertebrates like zebra fish carry out this remarkable regenerative process and why mammals have lost this ability might provide new ways to repair damaged human kidneys and dramatically extend and improve the lives of hundreds of thousands of patients with chronic renal failure.

Researchers at Brigham and Women's Hospital, Massachusetts General Hospital and the University of Pittsburgh have identified and characterized, for the first time, a progenitor cell in adult zebra fish kidneys that can be transplanted from one fish to another and generate new nephrons.

Now that this cell has been identified it may be possible to better understand how to increase its number and capacity to generate nephrons. Lead author, Alan Davidson, said, "We hope to eventually be able to cross species barriers and understand why similar cells, present in mouse and human kidneys during embryonic life, disappear around the time of birth".

The groups plan to continue studies on zebra fish and apply their data to mouse models and eventually humans.

The findings have been published in the journal *Nature*.

This is Wikipedia's entry about the journal.

Nature (journal)

For the U.S. magazine published in Baltimore between 1923–1959, see American Nature Association.

Nature, first published on 4 November 1869, is the world's most cited interdisciplinary science journal. Most scientific journals are now highly specialized, and *Nature* is among the few journals (the other weekly journals *Science* and *Proceedings of the National Academy of Sciences* are also prominent examples) that still publish original research articles across a wide range of scientific fields. There are many fields of scientific research in which important new advances and original research are published as either articles or letters in *Nature*. Research scientists are the primary audience for the journal, but summaries and accompanying articles are intended to make many of the most important papers understand- able to scientists in other fields and the educated general public. Towards the front of each issue are editorials, news and feature articles on issues of general interest to scientists, including current affairs, science funding, business, scientific ethics and research breakthroughs. There are also sections on books and arts. The remainder of the journal consists mostly of research articles, which are often dense and highly technical. Because of strict limits on the length of articles, often the printed text is actually a summary of the work in question with many details relegated to accompanying supplementary material on the journal's website.

In 2007 *Nature* (together with *Science*) received the Prince of Asturias Award for Communications and Humanity.

Keeping in mind that Wikipedia is open to editing anonymously, this information about the journal has the ring of truth to it. Of course, I researched it to the best of my ability. It looks like *Nature* is purely online now. I'm not scientifically oriented [except for Chronic Kidney Disease], but still found it fascinating. Take a look for yourself.

At The Heart of the Matter...

5/6/11   I've written about how important it is to be aware that you have CKD, especially when other medical issues arise. I was surprised that doctors had not already thought to take gender, height and weight into account when administering the dye during a heart test as suggested in the following article.

Kidney Damage After Heart Imaging Test

Women are at higher risk than men of developing kidney damage after undergoing a coronary angiogram, according to a Henry Ford Hospital study. Researchers found that women are 60 percent more likely than men to develop radio contrast-induced nephropathy (RCIN), an adverse side effect that causes kidney dysfunction within 24 to 72 hours after patients are administered an iodine contrast dye during the common heart imaging test. This is believed to be the first study in which researchers investigated whether gender played a role in patients developing RCIN after undergoing a coronary angiogram. RCIN is the third-leading cause of hospital-acquired kidney damage in the United States, after surgery and hypertension. The study is being presented Wednesday at the National Kidney Foundation's Spring Clinical Meeting in Las Vegas.

"While researchers say further study is needed to explain the gender risk, they theorize that a woman's size may be a factor," says Javier Neyra, M.D., an Internal Medicine resident at Henry Ford and the study's principal investigator. "Because men and women patients receive the same amount of dye during a coronary angiogram, it's possible the amount is just too much for a woman's body to handle given her smaller size," Dr. Neyra says. "Perhaps a woman's height and weight ought to be factored into the dosage."

Dr. Neyra says the contrast dye may cause the kidney's blood vessels to narrow, thus causing damage to the organ. He says women with a history of heart disease should consult with their physician about undergoing heart imaging tests using contrast dyes.

Contrast dye is used to improve the visibility of internal body structures during an imaging test. In a coronary angiogram, the dye enhances images of the heart's blood vessels and chambers.

In the Henry Ford study, researchers followed 1,211 patients who received a coronary angiogram from January 2008 to December 2009. Nearly 20 percent of women developed RCIN compared to 13.6 percent of men.

Dr. Neyra says other contributing factors in the gender risk could be age, hormonal levels and other chronic conditions. "We just don't know without further study," he says.

The article is from MNT.

I keep thinking of a line from a song in the play *Damn Yankees* as Nima sang it in her solo when she was a little girl: "You've got to have heart; all you really need is heart." Maybe it's not really all you need with CKD, but it sure helps.

A Drug for CKD?

5/10/11   Now that I've used all the information in my book, I've been cruising all over the web to see what's happening with our disease. I found the following article about a drug – yes, that's right, a drug – that just might be really helpful. I suddenly became very hopeful, despite my warning you not to get your hopes up about things that MIGHT be useful in slowing down CKD.

What caught me off guard about the current CKD treatment is the following statement from the article.
Despite the use of current treatments, many patients progress to renal failure.

I don't want to be one of those patients. I want this novel ap-proach drug to be developed before I need dialysis. I want kid-neys to be grown in labs before I need a new one. I want stem cell research to provide more ways to improve the lives of those on dialysis. But this article seems to offer the simplest solution: a drug to impede the slowing down of kidney function.

Until any one of the new advancements is ready for us, I'll contin-ue to stick to the renal diet, take the meds that have been prescribed and exercise for half an hour a day... while I hope.

Concert Pharmaceuticals Advances Novel Chronic Kidney Disease Treatment, CTP-499, in Phase 1 Clinical Study

Concert Pharmaceuticals, Inc. today announced it has made signif-icant progress advancing CTP-499, its novel anti-inflammatory, anti-oxidant, and anti-fibrotic agent for diabetic nephropathy and other forms of Chronic Kidney Disease, into clinical development. Based on encouraging preclinical results and successful formula-tion assessment in healthy volunteers, Concert has initiated a Phase 1 single ascending dose study of CTP-499 in healthy volun-teers. CTP-499, invented using Concert's DCE Platform™ (deuterated chemical entity platform), is a potential first-in-class treatment for Chronic Kidney Disease, a major and growing health problem.

"We are excited about the progress of CTP-499 and its potential to treat diabetic nephropathy and, more generally, Chronic Kidney Disease," said Roger Tung, Ph.D., President and Chief Executive Officer of Concert Pharmaceuticals. "Chronic Kidney Disease is a progressive disease that has become a major medical concern associated with substantial health care costs running to tens of billions of dollars per year in the US. Pre-clinical evidence that CTP-499 may protect kidney function and slow disease progression is encouraging. We look forward to advancing CTP-499 in clinical testing to evaluate its benefits in the treatment of diabetic nephropathy and other forms of Chronic Kidney Disease."

Diabetic nephropathy is associated with diabetes and is the leading cause of Chronic Kidney Disease in the US. Current standard of care for kidney disease is treatment with blood pressure lowering agents that affect the renin-angiotensin cascade, including Angiotensin Converting Enzyme inhibitors (ACEi) and Angiotensin Receptor Blockers (ARBs). Despite the use of current treatments, many patients progress to renal failure. There is a critical need for agents with novel mechanisms that further delay or prevent the decline of kidney function.

There is more technical information about this drug in the rest of the article.

Triple Digit Temperature Warning

5/14/11   Yesterday was our first triple digit day this year in sunny Arizona. It was also the day I decided to test drive cars in the middle of the afternoon. Not smart. But it did get me to thinking about what this kind of heat does to the kidneys. I found the following article, e-published last summer by DNA India. It explained quite a bit to me.

Heat-induced kidney ailments see 40% rise

Adversity is known to hit the down-trodden the most, but this summer, with its scorching sun and long list of heat-induced ailments, has spared no one. The latest development, say docs, is a massive increase in kidney failure and other kidney ailments, all caused by the heat.

A whopping 40% rise was noted in cases of kidney ailments in private hospitals, while government hospitals pegged the rise at 25%. Dr. HL Trivedi of the Institute of Kidney Diseases and Research Centre (IKDRC) said, "There has been a manifold rise in cases of heat-induced temporary kidney failures this month. Rapid loss causes the kidney's functioning to slow down, resulting in temporary or permanent kidney failure."

IKDRC confirmed about 25% rise in the number of cases this month. Priyadarshini Shah from IKDRC-ITS, said, "We usually get about 150 dialysis cases every day. However, a jump of about 25% has been noted this month." And this figure does not include more than half of the Total heat-induced temporary kidney ailment cases that are corrected either with oral medication or intravenous treatments.

Extreme heat causes rapid water loss, resulting in acute electrolyte imbalance. The kidney, unable to cope with the water loss, fails to flush out the requisite amount of Creatinine and other toxins from the body. Coupled with a lack of consistent water intake, this brings about permanent or temporary kidney failure, explain experts.

Dr. Shailesh Shah, a urologist with Kidneyline Hospital, said, "Due to heatstroke and water imbalance, an increase of about 20% has been noted in cases referred for dialysis, and of about 40% in heat-induced temporary kidney failure requiring intensive care." Complaints of kidney blockage due to stones and bleeding while passing urine, have also registered a rapid rise, informed Shah.

Commenting on this sudden increase, Dr. Himanshu Patel, a nephrologist, said, "The heat has also caused cases of Myoglobinuria – the presence of myoglobin in the urine, usually associated with muscle destruction, to increase."

Experts explain that symptoms of chronic kidney ailments and heat-induced kidney problems are different. Dr. Pranjal Modi, a kidney specialist, said, "Without adequate water intake, kidneys cannot function. Excessive perspiration and faster water loss due to exposure to the heat can cause diarrhoea, nausea and electrolyte imbalance, which often results in heat-induced kidney ailments. Here, a basic symptom of chronic kidney failure i.e. swelling is not present."

While this is not India, there are still parts of the country that will experience extreme heat. Be careful to avoid it as much as possible by staying in air conditioning, out of direct sunlight and being sure to drink your 64 ounces each day. Although heat induced kidney failure and CKD are not the same, both require that you drink enough water. To quote Dr. Modi from the article,

Without adequate water intake, kidneys cannot function.

The 24 Hour Urine Collection Revisited

5/17/11   I've just realized I'm a tweaker. Let me explain: I'm not a druggie, but rather someone who tries to finesse instructions in the way that best suits her.

I know, I know. You're asking yourself, "What is she talking about?" You see the title of today's blog and already know it's 24 hour urine collection day for me.

I woke up at 6:30 today after desperately trying to stay asleep and out of the bathroom until a more reasonable hour – say 7:30 – because I know I'll have to get up a little bit earlier than I did to-day to complete the 24 hour urine collection tomorrow. It IS a 24 hour test, after all. I just wanted to sleep a little later and didn't realize I could just start the collection period a little later until I read the 9/5/09 blog of Carolyn Cooper, MPH, RN.

This is the most complete explanation and set of instructions I've uncovered since I first began exploring this test and how to do it. If you remember, I've mentioned that sometimes the instructions your lab or doctor's office give you are simply not clear or thor-ough. I think we can thank Ms. Cooper for taking care of that problem for us.

24 Hour Urine Collection: How to do it and Why it's done

What's the Purpose of Urine Testing?

An incredible amount of information can be obtained from exam-ining a urine sample. In fact, over 100 different tests can be per-formed on a single specimen. Most of the time a simple "quick catch" specimen of urine (voided into a cup) is sufficient for a basic urine test. Urinalysis results may reveal problems with the body's electrolytes or hormones, the presence of infection, dehydration, evidence of microscopic blood (that can't be seen with the naked eye), drug levels, or problems with kidney function.

Why a 24-Hour Urine Collection?

A small sample of urine isn't always sufficient. In addition to blood tests, physicians will order a 24-hour urine collection if they have reason to be concerned about overall kidney function. This test typically focuses on creatinine clearance, sodium, protein, and urine osmolality. Other substances may be examined in a 24-hour collection; for example, hormone levels, urea nitrogen, or copper. The volume of urine that is voided during the 24-hour period also yields important information. The laboratory will make calculations based on your 24-hour (or 12-hour) urine collection that will help determine how well your body is clearing waste products via the urine. This finding will be compared to a blood test that measures how much of the waste products are circulating in your blood.

If your physician hasn't explained WHY he or she is requesting the 24-hour urine collection, ask for details. As a patient, being informed is one of your fundamental rights

Tips for Collecting Your 24-Hour Urine Specimen

A 24-hour urine collection is easy to mess up, and that can be very frustrating. Just one moment of accidentally forgetting to collect and save the urine during the 24-hours ruins the test, and the collection *might* have to start all over again . . .

Before the test

Your doctor's office will provide you with one or two brown plastic collection jugs and written instructions. Certain tests may require that urine be placed in a "double container" or that a preservative be added to the collected urine; you'll be given the supplies and containers appropriate for your test.

What you need from your lab or doctor's office

- Special instructions for the test and a lab sticker with your patient information to attach to the collection container(s).
- Collection container(s)–depending on the size of container the lab stocks–you may receive one or two of these jugs. They are made of heavy brown plastic, not just any container will do for this collection, so be sure to use the container(s) provided.
- Nice to have items–I'd ask for these if they don't offer them to you. **For men:** A plastic urinal to void into. **For women:** a plastic "nun's hat" to set in the toilet to collect the voided urine. If you don't have these items, it's okay to void into a bedpan, large plastic cup or bowl, etc. You will pour the collected urine into the brown collection container after each void, so it's nice to have something that pours easily.
- You'll also need a way to keep the collected urine cool during the collection period. One of the most common ways to do this is to set the brown urine collection jug in larger container filled with icy water (an ice bath). An ice chest (cooler) is another option. It's also possible to place the collection jug in the refrigerator, although there are many reasons to make this impractical.

When to begin?

Find out in advance when and where to return your 24-hour urine collection. This information will help you decide when to begin, because if the lab or physician's office isn't going to be open when you finish the collection, you'll have to keep the sample in a refrigerator, cooler, or in an ice bath until you *can* turn in your specimen.

It's often suggested that you begin a 24-hour collection first thing in the morning–but that is certainly not required. However, it *is essential* that you make note of the date and time that the specimen collection was started and stopped. This information will need to be recorded on the specimen container (and/or label).

Ready to start?

DO NOT save this first urine sample. The first time you empty your bladder you are flushing away urine that has been building up in your bladder for several hours or more. That hours-old urine will yield incorrect results if we collect it for our 24-hour specimen. We want to start with an empty bladder to collect only the urine our body makes during the 24-hour-period. **Record the start time and determine your stop time.**

All other urine during the 24-hours will need to be saved and poured into the collection jug. It's helpful to use the same bathroom all day long and post a note with the start/stop time to help remind you to collect all of your samples. Replenish the ice in the basin surrounding your collection jug from time-to-time in order to keep the specimen cool.

Ending the collection:

When the 24-hour-collection period is ending, make a last effort to urinate–even if you don't have the urge to "go," you will still be able to produce an ounce or two of urine. Make sure your collection jugs are tightly capped and labelled with your name, date of birth, collection date and start/stop times. (Note: If you weren't given a label for your specimen jug, *make one* and tape it securely to your jug.) Keep the specimen in the ice bath, cooler, or refrigerator until you are ready to return it to the lab or doctor's office. Place your specimen jug(s) in a sturdy plastic bag for easy carrying. (Your specimen will be just fine without being on ice while you return it to the lab or doctor's office—as long as you are not exposing it to heat for a prolonged period of time.)

What If…? Special Circumstances

- **You filled up the container the lab provided, but your 24-hour-collection is not yet complete.** Use a very clean glass or plastic container to continue collecting your urine. Your brown jug protects the collected urine from light–so if you have to use a transparent collection bottle, be sure to guard it from the light along with keeping it chilled. Using an ice chest would be a good strategy for you in this case–if that's not possible, cover the transparent container with a brown paper bag to protect it from the light. When you return your sample to the lab, keep the transparent container in a brown paper bag, or some similar technique to keep it protected from the light.
- **You have started the 24-hour-collection, but find you need to leave the house for several hours.** Take a backpack with you, a plastic bottle with a secure lid, and a large ziplock bag full of ice. This will allow you to carry your collection items discreetly. For ladies, a wide mouthed plastic container will allow you to urinate and pour the sample into your capped bottle. Your ziplock bag of ice will help keep your sample cool while you are on the go. I know this is a rather bulky idea, but the best I can come up with at the moment.
- **For patients with urinary catheters**. It would be preferable to start your collection with a fresh catheter bag in place–if that's not possible, it would be nice to clean the existing the current catheter bag and flushing the accumulated urine. Record this as your start time. During the remainder of the 24-hour-collection period, empty bag–at least remove the bag from the

catheter and give it a good rinse out. Begin your collection by completely emptying the foley bag into the brown collection jugs at regular intervals and keep the collection jugs in the refrigerator on in an ice bath just as anyone else would do. At the designated stop time, empty your collection bag for the last time.

- **Urine becomes mixed with feces or blood**. Do not empty any urine that has been contaminated by feces or menstrual blood into your collection jug. Make note of the time and stop the collection. Contact your lab or physician's office to inform them. In some cases, if enough time has elapsed (12 hours or more), your physician may give the go-ahead to stop the test early. Possibly, you may be asked to start all over again.

- **Patients who are incontinent (cannot hold their urine).** Certainly your physician may not realize (or remember) that a particular patient struggles with complete or partial incontinence issues. Perhaps the 24-hour-test will be impossible because of complete incontinence; perhaps they might recommend a bladder catheter for the test, or perhaps they might allow a shorter period of time (12-hours or thereabouts) for the urine collection.

- **"Oops! I didn't collect every void during the 24 hours!"** If you forget to collect all of your urine, the test results may be inaccurate. Talk to your lab or doctor's office before disposing of all that you've collected. If you have already completed at least 12 hours of the urine collection, mark down the time of the last urination and keep your container on ice or in the refrigerator as discussed later in this article. Talk to your physician's office or lab to let them know what you *have* been able to collect. They should be able to use your sample and calculate the important information based on the number of hours you have collected—but it's important that they know the correct number of hours when you turn in the sample. It's possible that you'll be asked to start all over again, but there's a good chance that they can use what you've collected and make adjustments to correctly calculate the results.

- **Why keep the urine specimen on ice?** The ice bath is just a technique for keeping the urine cool enough so that bacterial growth doesn't overwhelm your specimen. The ice bath should keep your specimen in the 40-45 degree Fahrenheit range as would your refrigerator. Keeping a 24-hour-specimen in the refrigerator is really awkward and inconvenient. Having your specimen container right there in the bathroom "on ice" is so much easier.
- **Other questions?** Call your physician's office or lab.

I realize I'd also forgotten the purpose of not collecting that first void of the morning until I read this blog. There's something about being reminded of what you know that's almost as satisfying as learning something new – which is what I hope you've done today.

Resources, Anyone?

5/20/11 In the final edit of my book, I realized just how many resources there are out there for us. I'll try to give you a taste of each in the next few blogs.

For example, today I did a plain old ordinary Yahoo search for 'CKD' and ended up at the following article from SpaceDaily.com of all places. They call themselves "your portal to space" and usually report on the newest developments in the space industry, but here we have our disease. Be sure to read the last paragraph at least twice.

Winding back the clock with kidney stem cells
Monash, Melbourne (SPX) May 20, 2011

Stem cell research courts both controversy and support in the community- depending on your viewpoint. Now, for the first time, scientists at Monash University's Immunology and Stem Cell Laboratories (MISCL) have shown that they can make human stem cells from healthy adult kidneys without working on human embryos, circumventing ethical concerns around this research.

This achievement will allow group leader Associate Professor Sharon Ricardo and her team to model genetic kidney diseases in the laboratory and tease out the mechanisms that control these difficult-to-treat disorders.

"We're taking human kidney cells and winding back the clock to make their early precursors," Associate Professor Ricardo said.

For the challenging project, which was published in the _Journal of the American Society of Nephrology_, the Monash researchers started with healthy adult kidney cells, which they reprogrammed back to an embryonic-like state, then compared these kidney stem cells with off-the-shelf embryonic stem cells, and showed that both could form different embryonic tissue types, with their genetic features preserved.

"These kidney cells had their slate wiped clean. Now that gives us the opportunity to change that kidney precursor into all kidney cell types," Associate Professor Ricardo said.

In collaboration with Professor Peter Kerr from Monash Medical Centre, the research team has now generated four stem cell lines from patients with polycystic kidney disease and Alport syndrome, two leading genetic kidney disorders.

"As these stem cells can divide indefinitely in a culture dish, we can make a limitless source of patient-specific stem cells, make kidney cysts and screen drugs on those cells," Associate Professor Ricardo said. "Our ultimate goal is to make off-the-shelf mature kidney cells that patients can use for drug testing and disease modelling."

Associate Professor Ricardo, who is approaching pharmaceutical companies to screen drugs on the kidney stem cells, believes that this personalised medicine approach will produce safer medicines in the future. But in the short-term, the Monash researcher plans to continue work on the kidney to study how environmental factors influence how kidney cells behave, tests drugs for their ability to reduce kidney cyst formation and cell proliferation, and better understand how genetic kidney disorders develop in the first place.

As someone who still isn't sure how she developed CKD, I'm really interested in the genetic aspect of this research. And environmental factors in developing the disease? What a marvelous idea – figure out what we're doing to our environment that ends up making us ill and stop doing it. As I see it, medical thinking has changed dramatically in the last few years.

Let's Hear It for The Vegetarians!

5/24/11 In my book, **_What Is It and How Did I Get It? Early Stage Chronic Kidney Disease_**, I discuss phosphorous a bit.

This is the second most plentiful mineral in the body and works closely with the first, calcium. Together, they produce strong bones and teeth. 85% of the phosphorous and calcium in our bodies is stored in the bones and teeth. The rest circulates in the blood except for about 5% that is in cells and tissues. Again, phosphorous is important for the kidneys since it filters out waste via them. Phosphorous balances and metabolizes other vitamins and minerals including vitamin D which is so important to CKD patients. As usual, it performs other functions, such as getting oxygen to tissues and changing protein, fat and carbohydrate into energy.

Be aware that kidney disease can cause excessive phosphorus. And what does that mean for Early Stage CKD patients? Not much if the phosphorous levels are kept low. Later, at Stages 4 and 5, bone problems including pain and breakage may be endured since excess phosphorous means the body tries to maintain balance by using the calcium that should be going to the bones. There are other consequences, but this is the one most easily understood.

Milk and dairy products contain phosphorous, which is why I'm limited to 4 ounces daily. Other foods that I, for one, need to limit or avoid due to their high phosphorous level are colas, peanut butter (which I, unfortunately, had just discovered much to my delight before being diagnosed), nuts, and cheeses.

To give you an idea why, my phosphorous limit per day is 800 mg. Two pancakes contain 476 mg. or well over half my daily allotment. Although both IHOP and Village Inn now make their pancakes from scratch, it's very rarely that I spend so much of my phosphorous allotment on them.

Today, I found the following article on Bioscholar.com which is fast becoming one of my favorite sites for Chronic Kidney Disease updates. I bolded what I considered new information – well, that is, new to me.

Vegetarian diet helps kidney disease patients stay healthy
Friday, December 24th, 2010

Phosphorous levels plummet in kidney disease patients who stick to a vegetarian diet, according to a study appearing in an upcoming issue of the *Clinical Journal of the American Society Nephrology* (CJASN). The results suggest that eating vegetables rather than meat can help kidney disease patients avoid accumulating toxic levels of this mineral in their bodies.

Individuals with kidney disease cannot adequately rid the body of phosphorus, which is found in dietary proteins and is a common food additive. Kidney disease patients must limit their phosphorous intake, **as high levels of the mineral can lead to heart disease and death.** While medical guidelines recommend low phosphorus diets for patients with Chronic Kidney Disease (CKD), phosphorus content is not listed on food labels.

Sharon Moe, and her colleagues studied the effects of vegetarian and meat-based diets on phosphorous levels in nine patients with CKD. Patients followed a vegetarian or meat-based diet for one week, followed by the opposite diet two to four weeks later. Blood and urine tests were performed at the end of each week on both diets.

Despite equivalent protein and phosphorus concentrations in the two diets, patients had lower blood phosphorus levels and decreased phosphorus excretion in the urine when they were on the vegetarian diet compared with the meat-based diet. While the investigators did not determine the reason for this difference, a grain-based diet has a lower phosphate-to-protein ratio and much of the phosphate is in the form of phytate, which is not absorbed in humans.

The authors concluded that their study demonstrates that the source of protein in the diet has a significant effect on phosphorus levels in patients with CKD. **Therefore, dietary counseling of patients with CKD must include information on not only the amount of phosphorous but also the source of protein from which it derives.**

"These results, if confirmed in longer studies, provide rationale for recommending a predominance of grain-based vegetarian sources of protein to patients with CKD. This diet would allow increased protein intake without adversely affecting phosphorus levels," the researchers wrote.

What Did You Say Phosphorous Is?

5/31/11   I've discussed phosphorus before but another point of view, or another way of explaining it, is always helpful. As usual, you benefit from my research. I especially like the substitutions for high phosphorous content foods in The National Kidney Foundation's Phosphorous Fact Sheet. I've reproduced most of the Fact Sheet here.

What is phosphorus?

Phosphorus is a mineral found in your bones. Along with calcium, phosphorus is needed for building healthy strong bones, as well as keeping other parts of your body healthy.

Why is phosphorus important to you?

Normal working kidneys can remove extra phosphorus in your blood. When you have Chronic Kidney Disease (CKD) your kidneys cannot remove phosphorus very well. High phosphorus levels can cause damage to your body. Extra phosphorus causes body changes that pull calcium out of your bones, making them weak. High phosphorus and calcium levels also lead to dangerous calcium deposits in blood vessels, lungs, eyes, and heart. Phosphorus and calcium control is very important for your overall health.

What is a safe blood level of phosphorus?

A normal phosphorus level is 3.5 to 5.5 mg/dL.

How can I control my phosphorus level?

You can keep your phosphorus level normal by understanding your diet and medications for phosphorus control. Your dietitian and doctor will help you with this. Below is a list of foods high in phosphorus.

HIGH PHOSPHORUS FOOD TO LIMIT OR AVOID

Beverages:
ale
beer
chocolate drinks
cocoa
dark colas
canned iced teas

Dairy Products:
cheese
cottage cheese
custard
ice cream
milk
pudding
cream soups
yogurt

black beans
chick peas
garbanzo beans
kidney beans
lentils
lima
northern beans
pork ' n beans
split peas
soy beans

Other foods:
bran cereals

brewer's yeast
caramels
nuts
seeds
wheat germ
whole grain products

What are medications for phosphorus control?

Your doctor may order a medicine called a phosphate binder for you to take with meals and snacks. This medicine will help control the amount of phosphorus your body absorbs from the foods you eat. There are many different kinds of phosphate binders. Pills, chewable tablets, and powders are available. Some types also contain calcium, while others do not. You should only take the phosphate binder that is ordered by your doctor or dietitian.

What do I do if my phosphorus level is too high?

When your phosphorus level is too high, think about your diet and substitute lower phosphorus foods for a while. Talk to your dietitian and doctor about making changes in your diet and ask about your phosphate binder prescription.

I find this refresher, well, ummm, refreshing. Think about it and maybe try making just one change this week.

[The National Kidney Foundation took the time to thank the Council on Renal Nutrition for the development of the fact sheet.]

Not Enough Kidney Doctors?

6/2/11 We finished shooting a movie tonight. That leaves you really keyed up, too keyed up to sleep. Since it's almost Friday, I decided to spend that non-sleeping time looking for interesting new developments in the management of CKD.

That wasn't what I found at sciencedaily.com. It made me think. When I needed a different doctor in the same practice, there was one available although there were no women doctors in the practice. There were Indian doctors, Filipino doctors, and, oh yes, one with a stereotypical North American name. What if there were no doctor to transfer to? What if only the one U.S. citizen doctor was there?

My nephrologist already seems to be drastically overworked and tells me about all the calls he has to make, the time he spends in the hospital and the time spent with patients. What if he were one of the very few nephrologists available? Apparently, that's not as farfetched as you may think. Read the article.

Can America Stop the Kidney Brain Drain? US Medical Students Are Rejecting Kidney Careers, Review Finds

Kidney disease affects 1 in 9 US adults, and by 2020 more than 750,000 Americans will be on dialysis or awaiting kidney transplant. Despite this growing health problem, every year fewer US medical students adopt nephrology as a career, according to a review appearing in an upcoming issue of the *Clinical Journal of the American Society Nephrology (CJASN)*. The review by ASN Workforce Committee Chair Mark G. Parker, MD (Division of Nephrology and Transplantation, Maine Medical Center) and colleagues highlights the declining interest of medical students in the US in nephrology. The authors propose ways to increase interest in nephrology so the US trains a sufficient number of kidney professionals to provide the growing demands of this public health crisis.

Dr. Parker explains that, "in medical school, students primarily work with hospitalized kidney patients, whose care is the most complex and daunting. And many students believe nephrologists to be overworked and underpaid." Nephrology is actually higher paid than a number of specialties, including rheumatology and hospital medicine. In a survey completed by the American Society of Nephrology (ASN) in 2010, 95% of nephrology fellows indicated they are happy with their career choice.

Although talented international medical graduates have historically contributed substantially to the US nephrology workforce, it is increasingly difficult for international medical graduates to obtain visas for the US, and this compounds the problem created by decreasing US medical students' interest in nephrology.

"We must work together to find a way to develop, improve, and market what we know to be a rewarding, stimulating, and fulfilling career," said ASN Councilor Bruce Molitoris, MD, FASN, chair of the ASN's Task Force on Increasing Interest in Nephrology Careers (Indiana University School of Medicine, Nephrology).

ASN has begun to implement strategies to inspire interest in nephrology among US medical graduates. Dr. Parker explains that "ASN will help provide stimulating experiences for trainees, nurture outstanding educators, and use social media to encourage the next generation of students to learn about the importance of kidney disease and the satisfaction many nephrologists derive from improving kidney care."

ASN will improve efforts to recruit women and minorities, currently under-represented in the nephrology physician workforce. Gains were made by females, Hispanics, and African Americans entering nephrology fellowships from 2002 to 2009. However, the increases by Hispanic and African American nephrology fellows still trailed gains made by other medical subspecialties.

I have a suggestion. What if every CKD patient encouraged his or her daughter, son, niece, nephew, neighbor's child, co-worker's child and every other child he knows to become a nephrologist? We know not all of the kids will be interested, have the academic acumen or the aptitude to become a nephrologist, but how many will? At least, they'd know what a nephrologist is and maybe even talk to their friends about the profession. It's not perfect as a plan, but it's a start.

Caution: Lonely Can Be Harmful To Your Health

6/7/11   I had intended to do a blog tour – a romp through the different CKD blogs on the web – today but found myself stopped cold by this intriguing article from the online version of *The Economist*. I can remember that when I was a child, if I seemed overly quiet or sad, my mother would say to me, "Go play with your brother. You'll feel better." She was right, but I had no idea that we were actually encouraging my physical health each time I did that.

Now, as an adult, I've been told that CKD may lead to inflammation. I've got to admit that I've never been happier that I enjoy both being with people and by myself and, most important of all, can count on my two hands the number of times I've felt lonely. Who knew that was contributing to fighting my own CKD?

The reason loneliness could be bad for your health

SCIENCE has many uses, but it doesn't often produce handy pick-up lines. Recent work on the genetics of disease, however, suggests a way of opening a conversation with that solitary attractive stranger in a bar: loneliness can make you ill.

Lonely people, it seems, are at greater risk than the gregarious of developing illnesses associated with chronic inflammation, such as heart disease and certain cancers. According to a paper published last year in the *Public Library of Science, Medicine*, the effect on mortality of loneliness is comparable with that of smoking and drinking. It examined, and combined the results of 148 previous studies that followed some 300,000 individuals for an average period of 7.5 years each, and controlled for factors such as age and pre-existing illness. It concluded that, over such a period, a gregarious person has a 50% better chance of surviving than a lonely one.

Steven Cole of the University of California, Los Angeles, thinks he may know why this is so. He told the AAAS meeting in Washington, DC, about his work studying the expression of genes in lonely people. Dr Cole harvested samples of white blood cells from both lonely and gregarious people. He then analysed the activity of their genes, as measured by the production of a substance called messenger RNA. This molecule carries instructions from the genes telling a cell which proteins to make. The level of messenger RNA from most genes was the same in both types of people. There were several dozen genes, however, that were less active in the lonely, and several dozen others that were more active. Moreover, both the less active and the more active gene types came from a small number of functional groups.

Broadly speaking, the genes less active in the lonely were those involved in staving off viral infections. Those that were more active were involved in protecting against bacteria. Dr Cole suspects this could help explain not only why the lonely are iller, but how, in evolutionary terms, this odd state of affairs has come about. For inflammation is an antibacterial response.

The crucial bit of the puzzle is that viruses have to be caught from another infected individual and they are usually species-specific. Bacteria, in contrast, often just lurk in the environment (like tetanus), and may thrive on many hosts (as does bubonic plague, for example). The gregarious are therefore at greater risk than the lonely of catching viruses and Dr Cole thus suggests that past evolution has created a mechanism (the details of which remain unclear) which causes white cells to respond appropriately. Conversely, the lonely are better off ramping up their protection against bacterial infection, which is a bigger relative risk to them.

What Dr Cole seems to have revealed, then, is a mechanism by which the environment (in this case the social environment) reaches inside a person's body and tweaks its genome so that it responds appropriately. It is not that the lonely and the gregarious are genetically different from each other. Rather, their genes are regulated differently, according to how sociable an individual is. Dr Cole thinks this regulation is part of a wider mechanism that tunes individuals to the circumstances they find themselves in. Where it goes wrong is when loneliness becomes chronic, and the inflammatory response becomes chronic at the same time.

Before civilisation intervened, such chronic loneliness would have been so rare (because isolated individuals are so vulnerable to predation) that evolution would have ignored it. Now, paradoxically, the large population that civilisation makes possible means loneliness is commonplace— and with it consequences that natural selection, which is blind to the future, has not yet had time to deal with.

I don't know about you, but this got me to wondering if everything in the entire universe has an effect on your health. I've often suspected that's true and am more convinced now that articles supporting this theory seem to fall into my lap.

A Heart Disease Risk Reducing Drug?

6/14/11 I found the following last week and had to read it several times since it's just a bit technical. I find myself amazed at the medical breakthroughs and while I'm not in favor of taking medications per se, there are times when they can greatly enhance the chances of your having a healthy – possibly longer – life. The article is worth a read.

I am a little concerned that the pharmaceutical company that produces the drug was partially responsible for funding the research, but maybe that's not such a bad thing in this case.

Vytorin Lowers Heart Disease Risk in Large Study of Kidney Patients

The cholesterol-lowering drug Vytorin reduced the risk of heart disease among kidney patients by as much as 25 percent, according to the results of the largest kidney disease trial ever conducted.

"People with kidney disease are at a high risk of heart attack and strokes," explained study author Dr. Colin Baigent, a professor of epidemiology at the University of Oxford in the U.K. "But there are very few studies attempting to see how that risk can be reduced. In healthy people we know that lowering LDL, or 'bad,' cholesterol reduces the risk. But now this is the first study to show that lowering LDL among people with kidney disease reduces risk as well."

Baigent and his colleagues report on their research, which was funded in part by Vytorin maker Merck/Schering-Plough Pharmaceuticals, in the June 9 online issue of *The Lancet*. The findings were to be presented this week at the UK Renal Association and British Renal Society meeting being held this week in Birmingham, England.

Vytorin is a combination of Zetia (ezetimibe) and the statin Zocor (simvastatin). Yesterday, the U.S. Food and Drug Administration called for warning labels on Zocor because of an increased risk of muscle damage that is seen among patients taking the highest dose — 80 milligrams a day — of that drug.

Baigent noted that although statins alone are known to be effective at lowering LDL, one of the challenges of treating kidney disease patients is that they do not process such drugs well, rendering high doses of statins potentially toxic. However, by pairing a relatively low dose of the statin Zocor with Zetia, the team hoped to achieve the same LDL-lowering effect while using a much lower dose of a statin. "This is a rather neat trick," said Baigent, who struggled with kidney disease himself some three decades ago. "This combination produces the same LDL-lowering effect as would triple the dose of statin alone."

In this study, the authors focused on a pool of nearly 9,300 male and female Chronic Kidney Disease patients aged 40 and up (with an average age of 62). All were participants in the "Study of Heart and Renal Protection" (SHARP) study, which was conducted over a seven-year period at 380 hospitals spread across 18 countries.

Beginning in 2003, roughly one-third of the patients were already on dialysis at the study's launch. Nearly two-thirds were men, and none had a prior history of heart attack.

About half of the patients were randomly given Vytorin; the other half was given placebo pills.

Patients were tracked for a minimum of four years. The team recorded all instances of heart attack, stroke, vascular procedures, hospitalizations and side effects.

The results: The Vytorin group experienced 17 percent fewer major cardiovascular events, compared with the placebo group.

What's more, because about a third of the Vytorin group failed to take the drug all the time, the researchers calculated that, with 100 percent compliance, Vytorin would actually have lowered the risk for major cardiovascular events by roughly 25 percent.

"This finding has major implications, both for people who are on kidney dialysis, and also the larger group of people who have some stage of kidney disease but have not yet reached the stage where they need dialysis," Baigent said.

"So, this will have ramifications for many, many millions of people," he added, "given the estimated 10 percent of the population that has some form of kidney disease."

Dr. Robert Provenzano, chief of nephrology at St. John Hospital and Medical Center in Detroit, echoed Baigent's opinion. "Chronic Kidney Disease is an epidemic in the world," he said. "As other countries become 'Westernized,' we find the incidence of Chronic Kidney Disease and end-stage renal failure increases. We see this in India, and in China. We see this everywhere. So, this is a huge issue.

The problem though is that even though we've already identified the basic risk factors, so far most of the data concerning cholesterol and risk has been circumstantial or confounded by a lot of other problems," Provenzano noted. "But now the SHARP study has answered the question, and found that LDL, bad cholesterol, directly impacts acceleration of Chronic Kidney Disease. And they've found a way to get around the high side-effect profile of statins by combining them with another medication.

Now if you have kidney disease, this won't cure you per se," he cautioned. "But it treats the co-morbidities that can kill these patients. And that makes this finding extremely useful."

Payback and a Hormone

6/17/11 This is admittedly bizarre, but when I read today's article, I got to thinking about how we never really know when it's all
going to end for us. No one likes to think about that, least of all
someone with a chronic illness. Here's the article that got me to
thinking about payback.

**Hormone Linked to Death Risk in Those With Early Kidney
Disease**
Strength of the association with mortality surprised researchers

Patients with early-stage Chronic Kidney Disease are more likely to
die if they have elevated levels of a certain hormone, a new study
says. Endocrine hormone fibroblast growth factor 23 (FGF-23)
regulates phosphorus metabolism. It was known that levels of
FGF-23 increase as kidney function declines and that high levels of
the hormone are associated with increased risk of death in
patients with kidney failure. But little was known about how
elevated levels of FGF-23 affect outcomes of patients with early-
stage Chronic Kidney Disease.

This study looked at 3,879 patients with early-stage Chronic Kidney Disease. During a median follow-up of 3.5 years, 266 of the
patients died and 410 progressed to kidney failure. The researchers found that median FGF-23 levels were higher in these patients than in those who remained "event-free."

Patients with the highest levels of FGF-23 were 4.3 times more
likely to die than those with the lowest levels, according to the
study in the June 15 issue of the *Journal of the American Medical
Association*.

The researchers said they were surprised to find that high FGF-23
levels were more strongly associated with death than other factors, including cardiovascular disease and Chronic Kidney Dis-

ease-specific risk factors such as reduced estimated glomerular filtration rate (GFR, a measure of the kidney's ability to filter out and remove waste products) and proteinuria (excessive protein in the urine).

The reasons for the link between elevated FGF-23 levels and increased risk of death aren't known.

"If the results of the current study are confirmed and experimental studies support the hypothesis of direct toxicity of FGF-23, future research should evaluate whether therapeutic or preventative strategies that lower FGF-23 can improve outcomes," Dr. Tamara Isakova, of the University of Miami Miller School of Medicine, and colleagues said in a news release from the journal.

I hope I've given you plenty to think about during the weekend. Payback doesn't have to be drudgery. I've recorded books for the Blind and Visually Impaired, organized food and clothing donations, been a hospice volunteer and, of course, the acting in the films. I've enjoyed each experience, even as a hospice volunteer. Just keep it in the back of your mind and let the idea percolate.

Another Reason to Be Happy

6/21/11 This morning I found another reason for those of us with Chronic Kidney Disease to be happy. I know! It sounds ridiculous.

Now that that's out of the way, there's seemingly always been the suspicion that physical illness and depression were connected. However, which came first? We have sort of a chicken and the egg situation here. This article may help you understand the connection.

Depression May Increase the Risk of Kidney Failure

Depression is associated with an increased risk of developing kidney failure in the future, according to a study appearing in an upcoming issue of the *Clinical Journal of the American Society Nephrology (*CJASN). Approximately 10% of the US population will suffer from depression at some point during their lifetime.

Lead investigator, Dr. Willem Kop (Department of Medical Psychology and Neuropsychology at the University of Tilburg, the Netherlands) and colleagues studied 5,785 people from four counties across the United States for 10 years. The participants were 65 years and older and not yet on dialysis. They completed a questionnaire measuring depressive symptoms and a broad range of medical measurements, including estimated glomerular filtration rate (eGFR) and risk factors for kidney and heart diseases. The investigators examined whether depression predicted the onset of kidney disease or other medical problems in which the kidneys play a critical role.

According to the results, depression coincided with the presence of Chronic Kidney Disease (CKD) and was 20% more common in individuals with kidney disease than those without kidney disease. The study shows that depression predicted subsequent rapid decline in kidney function, new onset clinically severe kidney disease (or end-stage renal disease), and hospitalizations that were complicated by acute kidney injury. When the investigators corrected for the long-term effects of other medical measures, the predictive value of depression for hospitalizations with acute kidney injury remained high.

Take home message: "People with elevated depressive symptoms have a higher risk of subsequent adverse kidney disease outcomes. This is partially explained by other medical factors related to depression and kidney disease. But, the association with depression was stronger in patients who were otherwise healthy compared to those who had co-existing medical disorders such as diabetes or heart disease," explains Kop.

The investigators are currently analyzing which factors may explain the association with depression, which could include delayed seeking of medical care and miscommunications between patient and physicians and important biological processes associated with depression, such as the immune and nervous systems.

Since I am almost 65 years and not yet on dialysis, I'll use this as the excuse I've been looking for to remain a Pollyanna and laugh at my woes. How bad can they be? I'm not dead and that's worth a bunch of laughter. I always use laughter. It's sustained me in the very worst of times with dear ones' illnesses and now my own. As they used to say in some old commercial, "Try it, you'll like it."

Baby, It's Hot Out There!

6/24/11 With temperatures of 110 degrees and over here this past week, I got to thinking about why – as CKD patients – we're warned to be extra careful about this weather and, specifically, exercising in this weather. I wanted to see how this all came together so I hit site after site with the same result: dehydration is the culprit. Of course, then I hit site after site to see just why that was. I can define it and so can you, but there's always more, isn't there?

That's where WebMD came in.   I thought this article on their website did a really good job of explaining in a common language we can all understand. It also discusses babies and older people, which are not necessarily my target groups, but can come in handy should you happen to have a baby or older person in your life.

Keep in mind that as a CKD patient, you are limited to 64 oz. of liquid [or at least, I am] no matter how much you sweat. This amount also includes ice cream, milk, coffee, tea, juice, frozen fruit pops, jello – anything that is or once was a liquid. Let's not squander this fluid on perspiration; we need to keep it to help our bodies function.

Dehydration occurs when your body loses too much fluid. This can happen when you stop drinking water or lose large amounts of fluid through diarrhea, vomiting, sweating, or exercise. Not drinking enough fluids can cause muscle cramps. You may feel faint. Usually your body can reabsorb fluid from your blood and other body tissues. But by the time you become severely dehydrated, you no longer have enough fluid in your body to get blood to your organs, and you may go into shock, which is a life-threatening condition.

Dehydration can occur in anyone of any age, but it is most dangerous for babies, small children, and older adults.

Dehydration in babies and small children

Babies and small children have an increased chance of becoming dehydrated because:

- A greater portion of their bodies is made of water.
- Children have a high metabolic rate, so their bodies use more water.
- A child's kidneys do not conserve water as well as an adult's kidneys.
- A child's natural defense system that helps fight infection (immune system) is not fully developed, which increases the chance of getting an illness that causes vomiting and diarrhea.
- Children often will not drink or eat when they are not feeling well.
- They depend on their caregivers to provide them with food and fluids.

Dehydration in older adults

Older adults have an increased chance of becoming dehydrated because they may:
- Not drink because they do not feel as thirsty as younger people.
- Have kidneys that do not work well. [You don't have to be older to have kidneys that do not work well. We have CKD. Our kidneys do not work well.]
- Choose not to drink because of the inability to control their bladders (incontinence).
- Have physical problems or a disease which makes it:
    - o Hard to drink or hold a glass.
    - o Painful to get up from a chair.

o Painful or exhausting to go to the bathroom.
o Difficult to talk or communicate to someone about their symptoms.
o Take medicines that increase urine output.
o Not have enough money to adequately feed themselves.

Watch babies, small children, and older adults [and CKD patients] closely for the early symptoms of dehydration any time they have illnesses that cause high fever, vomiting, or diarrhea. The early symptoms of dehydration are:

- A dry mouth and sticky saliva.
- Reduced urine output with dark yellow urine.
- Acting listless or easily irritated.

Now that I know how dehydration can disrupt my life in ways I could do without, I'm happy to know
a.) why I feel this way and
b.) I can do something about it - just like I can do something about keeping dialysis a long time down the pike by watching the chang-es I've made in my life.

Pumping Synthetic Iron

6/28/11 One of the first problems I faced after being diagnosed was the fatigue I felt most of the time. My doctor prescribed iron supplements, but they didn't do the trick. Then he suggested intravenous iron on a regular basis. My gut rebelled.

The thought of being stuck with even more needles on a regular basis was despicable to me. I was already taking blood tests every six months for the CKD and others every three months to monitor my liver function. That's a lot of needles.

I took care of the problem by instituting rest periods for myself each day instead of the IVs. It seems it's a good thing I did that considering the findings discussed in this article from Friday's Drugs.com.

FDA Urges Reduced Doses for Anemia Drugs

Doctors should use the anemia drugs Procrit, Epogen and Aranesp more cautiously in patients with Chronic Kidney Disease, U.S. health officials said Friday.

The new warning comes in response to data showing that patients on these drugs face a higher risk of cardiovascular problems such as heart attack, heart failure, stroke, blood clots and death, the U.S. Food and Drug Administration said.

"FDA is recommending new, more conservative dosing recommendations for erythropoiesis-stimulating agents [ESAs] for patients with Chronic Kidney Disease," Dr. Robert C. Kane, acting deputy director for safety in the division of hematology products, said during a news conference Friday.

These recommendations are being added to the drug label's black box warning and sections of the package inserts, he said.

This is not the first time health risks have been linked to these anemia drugs. They have also been tied to increased tumor growth in cancer patients and may cause some patients to die sooner. Also, cancer patients have an increased risk of blood clots, heart attack, heart failure and stroke, according to the FDA.

Procrit, Epogen and Aranesp are synthetic versions of a human protein known as erythropoietin that prods bone marrow to produce red blood cells. The drugs are typically used to treat anemia in cancer patients and to reduce the need for frequent blood transfusions. Anemia also occurs in patients with Chronic Kidney Disease. Anemia results from the body's inability to produce enough red blood cells, which contain the hemoglobin needed to carry oxygen to the cells.

Currently, labels on these drugs say ESAs should be used to achieve and maintain hemoglobin levels within 10 to 12 grams per deciliter of blood in patients with Chronic Kidney Disease. These target levels will no longer be given on the label, the agency added.

Hemoglobin levels greater than 11 grams per deciliter of blood increases the risk of stroke, heart attack, heart failure and blood clots and haven't been proven to provide any additional benefit to patients, according to the FDA.

The new label says that for patients with Chronic Kidney Disease not on dialysis, ESA therapy can be started when the hemoglobin level is less than 10 grams per deciliter. However, the goal of treatment should not be to increase hemoglobin levels to 10 or more grams per deciliter. Treatment needs to be individualized for each patient, the FDA said.

For patients on dialysis, ESA therapy can start when the hemoglobin level is less than 10 grams per deciliter. But, if the hemoglobin level approaches or goes over 11 grams per deciliter, the dose of the drug should be lowered or therapy stopped, the agency said.

Doctors should prescribe the lowest possible dose needed to reduce the need for transfusions, the agency added.

Patients taking these drugs should read the information in the medication guide included with these drugs. They should also have frequent blood tests, which help doctors keep hemoglobin at safe levels. If patients have concerns about these drugs, they should consult with their doctor, the FDA said.

Amgen Inc., the maker of all three drugs, said in a news release that it backs the FDA action.

"Amgen supports the modified ESA prescribing information as it informs physicians of important safety information," Dr. Roger M. Perlmutter, Amgen's executive vice president of research and development, said in the news release. "The revised label also provides physicians with more individualized treatment guidance by distinguishing between patients undergoing dialysis as compared with those who are not on dialysis."

The U.S. Centers for Disease Control and Prevention estimates that more than 20 million Americans aged 20 and older suffer from Chronic Kidney Disease.

Frankly, yesterday and today have been fraught with one emotional or business associated frustration after another, a very unusual situation for me. But three years ago, I made a decision that was good for me, even if I made it for the wrong reasons. Maybe it's extended my life. Maybe it's helped to impede the progress of my disease. Maybe not...

Home, Sweet Home

7/1/11 So many articles of interest to CKD patients flew across my monitor this week that it was difficult to decide which one to bring to your attention. I went about my daily business as I pondered this. One part of that business is taking my blood pressure reading at home. Bingo! Guess which article won today's attention. Once again, thank you Bio-Medicine and HealthDay News.

Blood pressure readings logged over a 24-hour period on a portable home monitoring device appear more effective than blood pressure readings taken in a doctor's office for predicting whether patients with Chronic Kidney Disease will experience kidney failure or death. That's the finding of an Italian study that included 436 Chronic Kidney Disease patients who were not on dialysis.

In the study, each patient's blood pressure was measured multiple times while at a clinic over the course of two days. They were also given an ambulatory blood pressure monitor that took readings every 15 minutes during the day and every half hour at night over a 24-hour period.

At-home blood pressure monitors are believed to help overcome what's known as "white coat hypertension," in which a patient's blood pressure spikes because of stress and anxiety when visiting a physician's office. According to background information in the article, Chronic Kidney Disease patients are especially vulnerable to this.

Prior research has also suggested that nighttime blood pressure readings may be a better measure of a patient's actual blood pressure status because readings are taken when the patient is at rest and free of the physical and emotional stresses of everyday life that can have an impact on readings.

During an average follow-up of 4.2 years, 86 patients developed kidney failure and 69 died. There were also 63 non-fatal cardiovascular events and 52 deaths caused by cardiovascular problems.

Patients with the highest risk of kidney or cardiovascular problems were those whose daytime systolic (top number) blood pressure was 135 mm Hg or higher; those with high diastolic (bottom number) readings; those with nighttime systolic readings of 124 mm Hg or higher; and those with nighttime diastolic readings of 70 mm Hg or higher. All these readings were provided by the ambulatory device.

"In contrast, office [blood pressure] measurements … did not predict cardiovascular or renal events," the researchers wrote.

Apparently, home is more than a place you hang your hat. It's the place where the true you resides as evidenced by your blood pressure readings.

The Other Clearinghouse

7/5/11 We all know about the Publishers' Clearinghouse and how we can win prizes from it [or can we?]. The National Kidney and Urologic Diseases Information Clearinghouse is much more important to us as Chronic Kidney Disease patients, although it doesn't seem to be some-thing a lot of us are informed about. So today, I'm going to introduce you to each other via their Winter 2011 Kidney Disease Research Update. Reader, meet NKUDIC. NKUDIC, meet Reader. Get to know each other.

Report Calls for Increased Coordination of Federal CKD Prevention and Treatment Efforts

Increased coordination of federal health efforts would vastly improve Chronic Kidney Disease (CKD) prevention and care, according to a recent report from the National Kidney Disease Education Program (NKDEP), part of the National Institute of Diabetes and Digestive and Kidney Diseases (NIDDK).

"Current Federal efforts span a range of missions, including surveillance, professional, and patient education, outreach to high-risk populations, quality improvement, and delivery of, as well as payment for, CKD treatment," wrote NKDEP Director Andrew S. Narva, M.D., F.A.C.P., and co-authors in the May 2010 issue of *Advances in Chronic Kidney Disease*. "However, Federal agencies do not function as a comprehensive system or, indeed, as a system at all."

Medicare spends more than $49 billion annually to care for patients with kidney disease. The NIDDK, together with other National Institutes of Health Institutes and centers, currently funds a $523 million kidney disease research portfolio. Other federal organizations, including the Centers for Disease Control and Prevention, the Indian Health Service, and the U.S. Department of Veterans Affairs, also contribute major funds and resources directed at CKD prevention and care.

Despite these enormous efforts, the percentage of people with CKD receiving recommended care has remained unchanged for many years. Fewer than 35 percent of people with diabetes and CKD are getting eye examinations or tests to measure blood sugar control or blood lipids. Blood pressure control among CKD patients remains poor. And despite tests that show the kidneys are not adequately filtering blood, many people with CKD are not being diagnosed and therefore are not receiving care to slow CKD progression.

About 23 million Americans 20 years old and older have CKD. Associated with diabetes, obesity, and cardiovascular disease, CKD prevalence has dramatically increased during the past 30 years. CKD is enormously expensive to treat, representing more than one-quarter of Medicare expenditures.

The report cited Quality Improvement Organizations (QIOs)—tasked by Congress to improve the quality of Medicare services—as having the potential to make great strides in CKD care quality. Each state has in place a QIO that consists of a private contractor or nonprofit organization. A recent initiative, called Ninth Scope of Work, focuses QIOs on determining the rate of diabetes-related kidney failure, slowing CKD progression by ensuring CKD patients are getting high blood pressure medication, and encouraging the early placement of arteriovenous fistulas—the best long-term vascular access—for CKD patients starting hemodialysis.

Kidney Interagency Coordinating Committee (KICC)

The KICC, chaired by Narva, brings together representatives from nine Government agencies involved in CKD to communicate and coordinate activities across sectors.

"The barriers to achieving greater effectiveness begin with poor visibility," wrote Narva and co-authors. "Federal program managers experience difficulty in learning about, and staying abreast of, what other Federal agencies do related to CKD."

In response, the KICC developed an interactive, web-based tool that summarizes CKD-related activities from all nine KICC participating agencies. Called the KICC Matrix, the tool is available on the NKDEP website.

Recommendations

Among the report's recommendations are the creation of a cross-agency initiative to define CKD-relevant improvement measures, an assessment of current CKD clinical guidelines, the development of better kidney failure prediction tools, and the coordination of efforts to strengthen CKD educational materials for health care providers. The report also recommends looking for successful models of federal collaboration outside CKD prevention and care.

Medicare Agrees

7/8/11   On June 28th, I posted an article about the new realization that kidney patients were being over-medicated with synthetic iron when dealing with their anemia problems. I explained that this option [the synthetic iron, not the then as yet unrecognized over-medicating] had been suggested to me several times, but due to my abhorrence of yet another set of needles – it is administered intravenously – I decided to pass on the treatment and deal with the anemia via daily rest periods.

Apparently, this is an issue of great interest currently. Medscape just posted a Reuters Health Information article dealing with this issue in dialysis patients. While we are not yet dialysis patients, supposedly we may be eventually. In the meanwhile, I urge you to think twice and research three times should your nephrologist suggest synthetic iron treatments for you.

Medicare Proposes Change in Anemia Drug Usage
by Deena Beasley

LOS ANGELES (Reuters) Jul 04 – The Medicare federal health insurance program has proposed removing its requirement that kidney dialysis providers keep patient hemoglobin levels above a set minimum, which could lead to lower use of Epogen, the anemia drug sold by Amgen. The government health plan said last month that it had no plans to change its reimbursement terms for anemia drugs used to treat kidney patients.

But in a statement on its website on Friday, the agency proposed retiring a requirement that patients' hemoglobin, or red blood cell, levels be kept above 10 milligrams per deciliter.

It said such an action would be "consistent with revised U.S. Food and Drug Administration guidelines."

Last week, the FDA changed the labels for Amgen's Epogen and Johnson and Johnson's Procrit to call for lower dosing of the anemia drugs, which have been linked in recent years to safety concerns such as increased risk of heart problems.

"Clinicians should use the lowest dose of ESA (erythropoiesis stimulating agent) sufficient to reduce the need for red blood cell transfusions," Patrick Conway, chief medical officer at the Centers for Medicare and Medicaid (CMS) said in the statement. Amgen said it recognizes that the labeling for ESAs has changed, but it is concerned that the proposal would remove an important safeguard designed to protect dialysis patients from being undertreated.

The Medicare guidelines "should have a measure that protects patients from hemoglobin levels that fall too low," the biotechnology company said in an emailed statement.

Sales of the anemia drugs have declined steeply in recent years, but Amgen's Epogen, along with its second-generation drug Aranesp, and J&J's Procrit are still expected to generate around $6 billion in 2011 sales, according to data from Thomson Reuters Pharma.

The proposed change would apply under Medicare's quality performance standards for "bundled" payments to dialysis providers and would affect payment years 2013 and 2014, the agency said.

CMS projected that its payment rates for dialysis treatments would increase by 1.8 percent in 2012, representing projected inflation of 3 percent less a projected productivity adjustment of 1.2 percent. It also estimated that federal payments to dialysis facilities in 2012 would total $8.3 billion.

While Medicare traditionally covers just elderly and disabled Americans, kidney disease patients are an exception. The program covers all those with end stage renal disease under a decades-old law.

Medicare said it would accept comments on the proposed rule until the end of August and will respond to them in a final rule to be issued by November 1.

I want to remind you that I am not a dialysis patient, simply a moderate stage Chronic Kidney Disease sufferer, yet Epogen intra-venously twice a month was recommended for me. I made my decision about this for my own reasons, but only after I explored the option. Should it be recommended to you, you need to do the same. Our nephrologists try to keep us in as good kidney health as possible, try to keep us informed, and try to keep us up on the latest findings, but we are the ones in charge of our own health.

It's Not Your Fault

7/12/11 I knew it wasn't all my fault and I resented taking all the blame – although it's clear I'll still have to take the responsibility for this. For what? For being obese, of course.

I discovered this article via Twitter on today's *New York Times Health Blog*. While it may absolve those of us who are obese from blame, as mentioned, it's still our responsibility to watch our weight. Obesity can be a cause of Chronic Kidney Disease, even if indirectly.

When Fatty Feasts Are Driven by Automatic Pilot

"Bet you can't eat just one" (as the old potato-chip commercials had it) is, of course, a bet most of us end up losing. But why? Is it simple lack of willpower that makes fatty snacks irresistible, or are deeper biological forces at work?

Some intriguing new research suggests the latter. Scientists in California and Italy reported last week that in rats given fatty foods, the body immediately began to release natural marijuanalike chemicals in the gut that kept them craving more.

The findings are among several recent studies that add new complexity to the obesity debate, suggesting that certain foods set off powerful chemical reactions in the body and the brain. Yes, it's still true that people gain weight because they eat more calories than they burn. But those compulsions may stem from biological systems over which the individual has no control.

"I do think some people come into the world, and they are more responsive to food," said Susan Carnell, a research associate at the Columbia University Institute of Human Nutrition. "I think there are many different routes to obesity."

In the recent rat studies, by a team from the University of California, Irvine, and the Italian Institute of Technology in Genoa, the goal was to measure how taste alone affects the body's response to food. Among rats given liquid diets high in fat, sugar or protein, the ones who got the fatty liquid had a striking reaction: As soon as it hit their taste buds, their digestive systems began producing endocannabinoids, chemicals similar to those produced by marijuana use.

The compounds serve a variety of functions, including regulation of mood and stress response, appetite, and movement of food through the intestines. Notably, they were released only when the rats tasted fat, not the sugar or protein. The findings were published online last week in the proceedings of the National Academy of Sciences.

"The most surprising thing to most people, including me," said an author of the study, Daniele Piomelli, director of drug discovery and development at U.C. Irvine, "is the findings provide a window on how we relate to fatty foods."

Since fats are essential for cell functioning, Dr. Piomelli continued, "we have this evolutionary drive to recognize fat, and when we have access to it, to consume as much as we possibly can."

The finding that the signal to eat more fat is released from the gut offers hope for potential new diet drugs. A Food and Drug Administration committee already has rejected one diet drug that blocks endocannabinoids, called Acomplia in Europe, where it was later withdrawn because it had severe psychological side effects, including suicidal thoughts. The new research suggests that the focus might be shifted to endocannabinoids in the gut, which could alleviate side effects in the brain.

In the rat studies, the researchers injected a cannabinoid-blocking drug into the intestines of the rats and found that they lost interest in the fatty food. "The effect is remarkable," Dr. Piomelli said. "They are no longer interested in feeding. They stop completely. We were amazed."

A drug based on the research is still years away, but the findings offer practical advice to consumers about the powerful biological forces at play when they snack on fatty junk foods.

"We think we eat it because we like it, but it's not just because we like, but because we want it," said Dr. David Kessler, former head of the F.D.A. and author of the book "The End of Overeating" (Rodale, 2009). "It has a lot more to do with our brains and the feedback mechanism to our brains than we realize."

Other studies have shown that the body's brain reward centers are strongly affected by the foods we eat.

For example, when obese women were shown pictures of high-calorie foods, their brains showed greater activity in regions asso-ciated with anticipating reward than did the brains of normal-weight women. "Reward centers were activated just by saying the words 'chocolate brownie,'" said Dr. Carnell of Columbia.

The question is whether some people are born more responsive to certain foods, or whether a lifetime of overeating leads to brain and body changes that promote a stronger food response. To shed light on that issue, Dr. Carnell is conducting studies looking at normal-weight teenagers who have obese parents, and as a result are at risk for becoming obese themselves. "I'm interested in whether the brain is responding differently even before they be-come obese," she said.

Dr. Kessler notes that consumers need to be aware that the body's natural signals are often overwhelmed by the abundance of choices and messages about food, so they must be extra vigi-lant about healthful eating.

"The pull is very strong, and there is a biological reason why food has such power over us," he said. "It's a real struggle, and it's not just a question of being lazy or lack of willpower. But just because your brain is being hijacked, that doesn't mean you don't have a responsibility to protect yourself."

Hot as Hades

7/15/11   My fiancé has gotten into the habit of looking up the weather forecast on his super-duper telephone before we go to sleep. This is Arizona, ladies and gentlemen. We have a low of 103 degrees with a high of 110 this week, unlike July 2 when we hit 118.

The Irish Kidney Association posted this DaVita article on a really hot day. I was glad to learn something new from it [spraying your mouth with lemon water to keep yourself from drying out] and wondered if you might, too.

If you do decide to get your daily 15 minutes of vitamin D via direct sunlight, remember to do it in the early morning, before the heat hits – especially if you live in a climate like mine.

Seven Summertime Precautions for People with Kidney Disease

There are certain precautions that everyone should take during the sunny and warm summer months. If you have Chronic Kidney Disease (CKD), you'll need to take a few additional steps to protect your health in the summertime or when visiting warmer climates.

1. Go outside and get moving

Sunny summer days are ideal for going outside and exercising. If you have kidney disease, be sure to check with your doctor before starting a summertime exercise routine. Your physician can help you create an exercise plan that will support your health. Even if you feel tired at times, easy exercises may help you feel better. Walking and yoga are two activities that put only minimal stress on the body. To reap the benefits of having sunlight activate vitamin D in your skin, so spend 10-15 minutes in the sun before applying sunscreen.

2. Keep good fluid balance

Check with your dietitian or healthcare team for guidance about your fluid intake and whether it should be adjusted on days that you spend more time outdoors. Be careful of very cold beverages, which can cause stomach cramps. It's best to avoid drinking caffeine or alcohol or ingesting large amounts of sugar, as these can actually cause your body to lose more fluid. Try to stay cool by wearing a hat or a wet bandana around your neck to help control your thirst. [When I was teaching high school in NYC, the kids had to take their state exams in heat and humidity. We all used the bandana trick. Some of the students soaked their bandanas and kept them in the freezer overnight. Now that was VERY effective.] You might want to carry a small spray bottle filled with lemon water or mouthwash to spray your mouth when you are feeling dry.

3.   Save your skin from sun exposure

Everyone should wear sunscreen and apply it liberally. Unprotected sun exposure can cause skin damage. Use a sunscreen with an SPF of at least 15. Remember to reapply your sunscreen every two hours and also right after swimming or exercising. A water-resistant sunscreen will be less likely to come off if you swim or perspire. You can also protect your skin by covering up with a shirt, wearing a hat or sitting in the shade. You may want to soak up some sun before applying sunscreen to activate some of the vitamin D in your skin. Ten to 15 minutes is all it takes.

4.   Wear sunglasses

Sunglasses protect your eyes in the same way that sunscreen protects your skin from harmful sun damage. Your sunglasses should block at least 99% of UVB rays and 50% of UVA rays. Wraparound sunglasses and other styles that completely cover the eyes are best.

5. Protect your access if you go swimming

If you are on dialysis and have a vascular access — whether it's an AV fistula, a graft or a catheter — remember to cover it with a protective dressing when you swim. Ask your nurse which holds up best in water. For those with a central venous catheter (CVC), they should not submerge themselves and the CVC in the water at all. For people on peritoneal dialysis (PD), your healthcare team will show you how to properly clamp your PD catheter shut. The PD catheter should be immobilized to avoid trauma to or tension on the catheter while swimming. The dressing should be changed as soon as you're done with swimming. When going for a swim, do so in the ocean or a chlorinated pool. Avoid bodies of water that aren't chlorinated, such as ponds, lakes and rivers, which have a greater chance of hosting bacteria that can infect your access.

6. Eat healthy summer foods

Research shows that fruits and vegetables are important for good health, yet most people don't eat enough. Summer is the perfect time to fill your plate with kidney-friendly foods that are low in phosphorus and potassium. Remember to practice portion control as all fruits and vegetables contain some potassium. Here is a list of fruits and vegetables that can add color and flavor to your kidney diet:

Fruits	**Vegetables**
Blackberries	Carrots
Blueberries	Cauliflower
Cherries	Cucumber
Grapes	Eggplant
Peaches	Green beans
Plums	Lettuce
Raspberries	Onion
Strawberries	Peppers (sweet and bell)

Watermelon
(1 cup per day)

Potatoes (leached)
Radishes
Snow peas
Summer squash

Use these summertime ingredients to make delicious meals found on DaVita's website.

7. Plan your vacation to include dialysis

When you're on dialysis you can still enjoy a summer vacation. To accommodate treatments while you're away, pre-planning is the key to a successful trip. If you do in-center hemodialysis or home hemodialysis (HHD), ask your nurse or social worker how you can schedule treatments at a dialysis center close to where you'll be staying. Home hemodialysis patients dialyzing with the NxStage System One can take their portable equipment with them and continue HHD while they're on vacation if they prefer.

People on peritoneal dialysis can also take their equipment with them. Be sure to pack enough supplies to do your PD exchanges when you're away. You can also work with your supplier to have dialysate delivered to your destination. Start planning at least three months before your trip, and ask fellow patients for any tips on the DaVita Discussion Forums.

Summary

By taking a common-sense approach to summer, you can enjoy long, warm days while you support your kidney health. Taking a few summertime precautions — protecting your skin, staying hydrated, controlling liquid intake and planning a summer getaway — means you can have fun and remain healthy.

*'Fat A**' Doesn't Sound That Bad Anymore*

7/19/11   'Fat A**' used to be a terrible insult. Nowadays, 'Fat Middle' is worse; it's life threatening. If you've read my book, you know I'm medically obese. If you've seen my picture, you know I look a little chubby. [Isn't that called 'some extra pounds to love'?] Now I find out I'm in danger of shortening my life since those extra pounds are all around my middle – the worst place for my health, especially since I have Chronic Kidney Disease. Again, from my book, once you have our disease, it's going to affect other areas of your health for the rest of your life. This article explains.

Kidney patients with higher waistline apparently face doubled risk of Death

Kidney disease patients wary of their waist size may be concerned for the good. As per a study led by Loyola University Health System scientists, patients suffering from kidney problems who have a large waist size appear to face a higher risk of death.

Apparently, waist circumference was largely associated to mortality than another common measure of obesity namely body mass index (BMI). BMI is a height-to-weight ratio while waist circumference is simply the measure of the abdominal mass. Investigators observed information from 5,805 kidney patients aged 45 years and older and who enrolled for a study known as Reasons for Geographic and Racial Differences in Stroke (REGARDS). They all faced surveillance for an average of 4 years where it was found that 686 participants died during the course of the study.

The median BMI of the patients who passed away was 29.2 which were seemingly lower than the BMI of the patients who were alive. Contrarily, the mean waist circumference of the patients who faced demise seemed to be 40.1 inches which is apparently higher than the patients who survived and had a waistline of 39.1 inches.

Analysts drew a comparison between kidney disease patients with large waist size to normal waistline counterparts. The BMI and other risk factors were suitably adjusted and it came to fore that those women with a waist size equal to or higher than 42.5 inches and men with 48 inches or larger waist size supposedly faced a higher chance of dying. This was not the case for those who had a slimmer waistline which was almost 31.5 inches for women and 37 inches for men.

The scientists conclude that BMI may not be sufficient to gauge mortality risks linked to fat. This is mainly as BMI is inclusive of many factors like muscle mass and abdominal fat. Paradoxically, waist circumference is the measure of only the abdominal adiposity and may therefore be an essential tool to comprehend death risk linked with obese Chronic Kidney Disease adults specifically when used collectively with BMI.

Another thing I discussed in **What Is It and How Did I Get It? Early Stage Chronic Kidney Disease** is how complicated the formula for measuring BMI is. As a math repelled person, I had to resort to online BMI calculators. These are really a great help; I was just annoyed I couldn't do it manually. Now, there seems to be no reason to use this.

Just grab a tape measure and measure your waistline. You can even do it without a tape measure if you only have a ruler. Wrap a string, ribbon or cord around your waist and then measure its length with your ruler. But keep in mind as you're measuring that this is still a theory – one I like – but one of many.

Just When We Thought We Understood

7/22/11   I don't want to have Chronic Kidney Disease. I have no emotional need to be a patient. But when I read the following blog by England's Dr. Dan Brett yesterday, all I kept thinking is, "I don't want to be that part of that 1%." If only there were a way to predict who would be, I'd have to agree with him. BUT there isn't, so I don't [although I did find his thoughts comforting].

Prior to 2006, a gentle upward drift in creatinine, as patients grew older, was considered to be a part of natural ageing. It wasn't as if my patients were regularly popping their clogs due to end stage renal failure, leaving me berating myself for not checking their eGFR or urine protein/creatinine ratio. Notes might have been annotated with a 'mild renal impairment' code by the most diligent of us, but kidneys, on the whole, were strictly foodstuff or organs for connoisseurs and specialists.

Then 'Chronic Kidney Disease', with all it's [sic] stages, was invented – and added to QoF [I had to look that one up: Quality and Outcomes Framework]. With money attached, it immediately became 'important'. Literally hundreds of unsuspecting, asymptomatic patients – mainly elderly, have been dragged in to be given their bad news – cluttering up my waiting room, having umpteen blood tests and urine tests.

Doctor: "You've got stage 3 Chronic Kidney Disease, Mrs Miggins, requiring that we mount an immediate renin-angiotensin blockade, get you on a statin…"

Mrs Miggins: "Oh dear – stage 3 already you say! How long have I got…?"

Patients have been scared witless – terrified that a transplant/ dialysis /imminent death awaits them. [This is exactly why I wrote ***What Is It and How Did I Get It? Early Stage Chronic Kidney Dis-***

ease.] Renal referrals have rocketed and what exactly has been achieved? After four years of industrious GP QoFing, where is the evidence that managing Chronic Kidney Disease is of benefit? According to published studies, only 1% of patients with the stage 3 Chronic Kidney Disease label will progress to end stage renal failure in the next eight years. With these small percentages we need to treat thousands of patients each year to potentially make any difference at all! But doesn't managing Chronic Kidney Disease reduce deaths from ischaemic heart disease, I hear you say? Nope – kidding yourself again – evidence is distinctly lacking. Hoerr's Law rightly asserts that – 'It is difficult to make an asymptomatic patient feel better.'

Or put another way, in the words of our godfather – Hippocrates – 'To do nothing is also a good remedy'.

I have no intention of stopping my treatment, but whenever that panic starts to creep into my heart, I'll have this blog to quell it immediately. I'm pretty good about being rational concerning my Chronic Kidney Disease, but I'm also human and those what-ifs can make the teeniest little bit of headway when I'm feeling low. Maybe you can use it, too.

Another Job for the Kidneys

7/26/11   Our kidneys are very busy organs, indeed. They produce urine, remove potentially harmful waste products from the blood, aid in the maintenance of the local environment around the cells of the body, help to stimulate the production of red blood cells, regulate blood pressure, help regulate various substances in the blood [for example, potassium, sodium, calcium and more], help to regulate the acidity of the blood, and regulate the amount of water in the body. Mind you, these are just their main jobs. I haven't even mentioned their minor ones. And now, scientists have discovered they perform yet another function for us.

Science Daily ran the following article on the 21st of this month.

Kidney Dopamine Regulates Blood Pressure, Life Span

The neurotransmitter dopamine is best known for its roles in the brain — in signaling pathways that control movement, motivation, reward, learning and memory.

Now, Vanderbilt University Medical Center investigators have demonstrated that dopamine produced outside the brain — in the kidneys — is important for renal function, blood pressure regulation and life span. Their studies, published in the July *Journal of Clinical Investigation*, suggest that the kidney-specific dopamine system may be a therapeutic target for treating hypertension and kidney diseases such as diabetic nephropathy.

Previous studies had suggested a role for dopamine in regulating kidney function and total body fluid volume, "but how that mechanism works was not clear," said Raymond Harris, M.D., chief of the Division of Nephrology and Hypertension at Vanderbilt.

To explore dopamine's role in the kidney, Harris and Ming-Zhi Zhang, M.D., assistant professor of Medicine at Vanderbilt, eliminated kidney-specific dopamine production in mice (by knocking out a dopamine-generating enzyme only in the kidney) and studied the outcome.

They found that mice lacking kidney dopamine had high blood pressure at baseline and became more hypertensive when they consumed a high-salt diet, suggesting they may be a good model of salt-sensitive (essential) hypertension, Harris said. Alterations in the kidney dopamine system may predispose individuals to hypertension, he noted.

The investigators also showed that elimination of kidney dopamine increased renin production, which activates the angiotensin II system to increase salt and water reabsorption — and produce hypertension.

"These animals retain salt and water when they don't have sufficient dopamine production in the kidney," Harris said. "Our studies highlight this whole other hormonal system that appears to balance or put the brakes on the renin-angiotensin system."

Currently, the renin-angiotensin system is the major target for treating Chronic Kidney Diseases. Discovering another target — the kidney dopamine system — is exciting, the researchers said. They are exploring whether specific drugs that enhance the kidney dopamine system are effective in blocking hypertension and treating progressive kidney diseases.

The investigators predicted changes in kidney function in the mouse model, but they were "very surprised" to discover that the modified mice only lived about half as long as normal mice (15 months versus 30 months). They found increases in stress-related proteins in the kidney, heart and vasculature, suggesting that elimination of kidney dopamine causes systemic effects, Harris said.

"This kidney-specific dopamine system is not only important for kidney function and blood pressure regulation, but also for the overall health of the animal," Harris said. "If the dopamine system in the kidney is altered, the animals have a markedly shortened life span."

Once before I ran across research that suggested Chronic Kidney Disease could be treated with a drug. Now here it is again. For someone who felt hopeless when I first heard my diagnosis, I am becoming more and more hopeful with each round of research I do.

It's – Almost – Not Science Fiction Anymore!

7/19/11   Included in the blogroll of this blog is the American Society of Nephrology. Personally, I'm thankful this organization was one of the first to acknowledge my blog. As a Chronic Kidney Disease patient, I'm thankful they exist to keep us updated on the latest findings about our disease [among other things]. This is the largest organization to deal with kidney disease. That would explain why I periodically look at their site to see if there's anything to share with early stage patients.   On Wednesday, their tweet referred to an article that could make kidney patients who are dreading eventual dialysis cry – for joy, that is. I freely admit I am one of those.

Reprogrammed kidney cells could make transplants and dialysis things of the past

- Patients' own kidney cells can be reprogrammed and used as therapy against kidney disease
- Cells can easily be collected from the urine
- 88,000 patients are waiting for a kidney transplant in the United States, and they wait for an average of 3 to 5 years

Approximately 60 million people across the globe have Chronic Kidney Disease, and many will need dialysis or a transplant. Breakthrough research published in the *Journal of the American Society Nephrology* (JASN) indicates that patients' own kidney cells can be gathered and reprogrammed. Reprogramming patients' kidney cells could mean that in the future, fewer patients with kidney disease would require complicated, expensive procedures that affect their quality of life.

In the first study, Sharon Ricardo, PhD (Monash University, in Clayton, Australia) and her colleagues took cells from an individual's kidney and coaxed them to become progenitor cells, allowing the immature cells to form any type in the kidney. Specifically, they inserted several key reprogramming genes into the renal cells that made them capable of forming other cells.

In a second study, Miguel Esteban, MD, PhD (Chinese Academy of Sciences, in Guangzhou, China) and his colleagues found that kidney cells collected from a patient's urine can also be reprogrammed in this way. Using cells from urine allows a technology easy to implement in a clinic setting. Even better, the urine cells could be frozen and later thawed before they were manipulated.

If researchers can expand the reprogrammed cells—called induced pluripotent stem cells (iPSCs)—and return them to the patient, these IPSCs may restore the health and vitality of the kidneys. In addition to providing a potentially curative therapy for patients, the breakthroughs might also help investigators to study the causes of kidney disease and to screen new drugs that could be used to treat them.

In an accompanying editorial, Ian Rogers, PhD (Mount Sinai Hospital, in Toronto, Ontario, Canada) noted that "together, these two articles demonstrate the feasibility of using kidney cells as a source of iPSCs, and efficient production of adult iPSCs from urine means that cells can be collected at any time."

Just as exciting, the ease of collection and high frequency of reprogramming described in these articles may help improve future therapies in many other areas of medicine.

Be sure to take into account the "potentially," "could mean," and "if" included in the article. This is not a fait accompli, but we're certainly closer to avoiding dialysis than we've ever been before. [not so silent happy dance in front of the computer]

They're Connected

8/2/11 If you've had the chance to read ***What Is It and How Did I Get It? Early Stage Chronic Kidney Disease***, you'll know there was a time when I had a low potassium count. That's when the nephrologist gave me a list of low, medium and high potassium foods and told me to eat more of the high potassium foods. There was no accompanying explanation for why as far as I can remember.

Then I found this in BrightHub.com's February 13th article "The Importance of the Potassium and Sodium Balance."

When there is potassium and sodium balance, cells, nerves and muscles can all function smoothly. With an imbalance, which is almost always due to both an excess of sodium, and a deficiency of potassium, a set of reactions occurs leading to high blood pressure and unnecessary strain on blood vessels, the heart and the kidneys. Research has shown that there is a direct link between chronic levels of low potassium and kidney disease, lung disorders, hypertension and stroke.

Now that you and I know how the two minerals interact, the following article makes sense. As a matter of fact, it makes me wonder why these guidelines were not put into place a long time ago. Applause for Nurses.com, please! They're the ones who have explained in terms we can all understand why the Dietary Guidelines for Americans needed to be changed. Now, if only I could figure out how we became such a sodium loving culture in the first place....

Study: Sodium, potassium both affect mortality

Americans who eat a diet high in sodium and low in potassium have a 50% increased risk of death from any cause, and about twice the risk of death from a myocardial infarction, according to a study.

Researchers with the Centers for Disease Control and Prevention, Emory University and Harvard University said the study is the first to examine, using a nationally representative sample, the association between mortality and people's usual intake of sodium and potassium. The study analyzed data from the National Health and Nutrition Examination Survey, a survey designed to assess the health and nutritional status of adults in the United States. Usual intake of sodium and potassium was based on dietary recall.

"The study's findings are particularly troubling because U.S. adults consume an average of 3,300 milligrams of sodium a day, more than twice the current recommended limit for most Americans," Elena Kuklina, MD, PhD, an investigator on the study and a nutritional epidemiologist with the CDC's Division for Heart Disease and Stroke Prevention, said in a news release.

"This study provides further evidence to support current public health recommendations to reduce sodium levels in processed foods, given that nearly 80% of people's sodium intake comes from packaged and restaurant foods. Increasing potassium intake may have additional health benefits."

The 2010 Dietary Guidelines for Americans recommend limiting intake of sodium to 1,500 milligrams a day for people 51 and older, African Americans and those who have hypertension, diabetes, or Chronic Kidney Disease — about half the U.S. population ages 2 and older. The dietary guidelines recommend that all other people consume less than 2,300 milligrams of sodium a day. In addition, the guidelines recommend that people choose more potassium-rich foods, advising 4,700 milligrams of potassium per day.

Sodium, primarily consumed as salt, is commonly added to many processed and restaurant foods, while potassium is naturally present in many fresh foods. For example, cheese, processed meats, breads, soups, fast foods and pastries tend to have more sodium than potassium. Yogurt, milk, fruits and vegetables tend to have less sodium and more potassium. Potassium-rich fruits and vegetables include leafy greens such as spinach and collards, grapes, blackberries, carrots, potatoes and citrus fruits such as oranges and grapefruit.

In general, people who reduce their sodium consumption or increase their potassium consumption — or do both — benefit from improved blood pressure and reduce their risk for developing other serious health problems, according to the researchers. They said adults can improve their health by knowing recommended limits for daily sodium intake; choosing foods such as fresh or frozen fruits and vegetables, unprocessed or minimally processed meat or poultry, low-fat milk or plain yogurt; asking for foods with no or low salt at restaurants, and reading the nutrition labels of foods before purchasing can improve health for all adults.

The CDC is working with public - and private - sector partners at the national, state, and local levels to educate the public about the health effects of sodium and to reduce sodium intake. The agency is also enhancing the monitoring of sodium intake and expanding the scientific literature on sodium and health.

Take Active Control

8/5/11   I have been explaining – in ***What Is It and How Did I Get It? Early Stage Chronic Kidney Disease*** and in my life – that taking active control of your Chronic Kidney Disease is an absolute necessity. Today, I ran across this press release that re-enforces my thinking, but remember this IS a press release.

Revolutionary Baseline E-Health Platform for Kidney Disease Launched Today by Shad Ireland Foundation Innovative Empowerment Tool Tackles Compliance, Potentially Saves Millions to U.S. HealthCare System
ATLANTA, Jul 21, 2011 (BUSINESS WIRE) –

Baseline, ..., a technology driven e-health platform designed to empower millions suffering from kidney disease, was officially launched today by the Shad Ireland Foundation. The online platform, a proprietary technology funded by a grant from AMGEN Medical Education, offers solution-based tools and health care resources for individuals via the internet and mobile devices. When utilized, the Baseline solution has been shown to improve outcomes and compliance while helping patients create stability and rehabilitation in their lives.

Created in response to the rising number of individuals suffering from kidney disease and its precursors — diabetes, obesity and high blood pressure — Baseline's comprehensive solutions educate, engage and empower the end user to take an active role in their health care. Individuals with Chronic Kidney Disease, (CKD), End Stage Kidney Disease, (ESRD), and kidney transplant recipients can easily monitor their health, tracking key indicators, nutrition and exercise, plus receive lifesaving information regarding the disease 24 hours a day.

"People lose hope and let go of their life goals when given a kidney disease diagnosis," said Shad Ireland, Executive Director of the

Shad Ireland Foundation. "We want to show them that a diagnosis is not a death sentence. With Baseline, our goal is to offer inspiration and tools for healthy living. Using my 29 years of successfully living with this disease and other success stories as examples, we can inspire, engage, educate and empower people with kidney disease to stabilize their health and achieve their dreams. Baseline has the potential to help millions of people live a better life. I'm living proof."

Results Through Improved Outcomes & Compliance

Modeled after Ireland's positive results in living with CKD, and extensive medical research on compliance, Baseline is the first-ever technology driven solution targeted to the renal community. A potential answer to issues of compliance, outcomes and quality of life, Baseline promotes stability by managing key indicators, including nutrition and exercise.

Patients can track lab values, and other indicators working in tandem with their doctors to take an active role in their healthcare by controlling the disease. Baseline is also the first resource designed to address the government-mandated conditions for coverage for patients awaiting kidney transplants, providing critical information and tools to those in need.

While the average American with Chronic Kidney Disease is hospitalized four to six times per year, since taking active control of his healthcare, Ireland, a triathlete best known for successfully completing over 20 Ironman competitions, has only been hospitalized three times in the past nine years. An active athlete, Ireland is currently riding stages of some of the sport of cycling's toughest competitions as part of his Take on the Tour Project, ... , including the Tour of Colorado and the Tour of Utah, as well as running this year's New York City Marathon. Ireland is an example of the positive results that are possible from an engaged and educated patient.

"What Shad has shown us with the new Baseline tool is that physical activity and regular, structured, measured, and quantifiable exercise are really the keys to getting kidney disease under control," said Dr. Tom Pintar, Board Certified Nephrologist and Medical Advisor to the Baseline program. "In addition, this e-health platform has the potential to improve overall quality and quantity of life, which over time can lower healthcare costs. Considering our current health care crisis, it's an important issue for our country and around the world today."

New Technology Creates Easy to Use Compliance Tool

The proprietary Baseline e-health platform, created in cooperation with some of the best and brightest minds in technology, is based on Shad Ireland's life experiences. Working with the team, Ireland shared the lessons learned from his 29 years of dialysis to help create a comprehensive tool for other kidney disease patients and those predisposed to developing a kidney diagnosis.

"Shad has drawn from his life experience to create an intelligent application of technology and media that offers life enhancing resources and information to people who need it," said Rey Ramsey, Chairman for Technet. "Baseline offers the best solution for healthcare outcomes and compliance. I believe it will make a significant difference and improve the quality of life for patients living with kidney disease."

The Baseline e-health platform also includes a social component providing patients an opportunity to interact and share information. The groundbreaking platform is a benchmark case study of how non-profit and for profit companies can combine forces for the common good of the patient and is a cost-effective tool that uniquely engages the user while also providing resources to empower individuals to take a more active role in their health care.

A Salty Dilemma

8/9/11   Just as I realize all these years of watching the sodium content of foods has left me with a distinct dislike for salty foods – you know, the ones with the most flavor – the salt controversy comes to the fore. I think you'll need to take this information with a grain of salt [Sorry, couldn't resist.] in light of other recent posts about sodium and health despite the fact that this is Campbell Soup, for heaven's sake! The article is long, but clearly presents both sides of the controversy.

Campbell Soup Increases Sodium As New Studies Vindicate Salt

In February 2010, Campbell Soup announced that it would reformulate over 60% of its condensed soups to reduce the sodium content of 23 of them up to 45%. With high salt diets having been previously linked to cardiovascular disease in medical studies, health advocates were delighted. Last week the company's CEO-elect, Denise Morrison, made another announcement, this time a somewhat more alarming one. The company is putting the salt back in. With Campbell's soup sales sliding in recent times, Morrison believes that lower salt levels have translated to lower taste for their customers, and that the tweaked offerings may have been responsible for the flagging financials. The company hopes to tempt soup-lovers back by increasing sodium levels up to about 650mg per serving (they had been brought down from 800mg to 480mg) in many of the cans in their Select Harvest line.

Campbell's new strategy appears all the more startling in light of the fact that the US Department of Agriculture's 2011 Dietary Guidelines couldn't be any clearer on the point that, as a nation, we need to step away from the salt shaker. "Virtually all Americans consume more sodium than they need," it says.

According to research by the U.S. Centers for Disease Control and Prevention, the average American adult currently consumes

3,436 mg of salt a day. With an estimated 75% of our salt intake coming from processed and packaged foods, the USDA guidelines go on to add: "An immediate, deliberate reduction in the sodium content of foods in the marketplace is necessary to allow consumers to reduce sodium intake to less than 2,300 mg or 1,500 mg per day [for those aged 51+, all African Americans, plus anyone with hypertension, diabetes, or Chronic Kidney Disease] now."

Faced with pressure to ease up on sodium, big players in the food industry, such as Kraft Foods, Heinz and Unilever have responded by recently joining the National Salt Reduction Initiative (NSRI), which aims to slash salt content in retail and foodservice throughout the country by 20% in five years

Again, next to this, Campbell's renegade approach *seems* irresponsible. Surely the company should continue to encourage a healthier consumer base which, presumably, will stick around longer to enjoy its products? This is especially since research shows that our perceptions of saltiness and taste intensities can change over a relatively short period of time. In plain speak, this means that if Campbell's perseveres with the lower salt offerings and convinces its customers to do the same, diners will quickly grow accustomed to the more modestly seasoned soups.

But, maybe we shouldn't be so quick to condemn Campbell's new strategy. After all, recently published pro-sodium studies suggest that food manufacturers across the board should actually be following Campbell's lead. Contrary to everything we've been previously fed, a high-profile scientific paper by The Cochrane Library, came to the following straight-stalking (sic) conclusion: "cutting down on the amount of salt has no clear benefits in terms of likelihood of dying or experiencing cardiovascular disease".

The paper, published last week in the Journal of Hypertension, reviewed seven studies, which in total included 6489 participants, a number which, the authors say, provides sufficiently reliable results. The study – led by Professor Rod Taylor from Peninsula College of Medicine and Dentistry in the UK, found no evidence to support the theory that a reduction in salt intake decreases cardiovascular disease or all-cause mortality in those with normal or raised blood pressure. Astonishingly, it also concluded that salt reduction could be detrimental to health. In people with congestive heart failure, salt restriction actually *increases* the risk of death from all causes, the paper claims.

If this all sounds a little sketchy to you, especially since salt has been demonized no end until now, there's more research to support the idea that we should give the tasty mineral a break. You might recall a perplexing study published in the May issue of the *Journal of the American Medical Association*. It surmised that people who eat *lower amounts* of sodium are *more likely* to die from cardiovascular disease and that, among those with normal blood pressure, sodium intake didn't lead to high blood pressure.

Certainly these pro-salt studies have created something of a media frenzy, and they have amassed critics aplenty. The May study was so riddled with problems and flaws it prompted Harvard researchers to deem its conclusions as "most certainly wrong." The main complaint was that most of the participants in the study were in their early 40s when the research began, and were only tracked for about eight years. This entailed that the population was too young to reliably determine how sodium intake could impact their long-term health.

As for the Cochrane Review, medical experts are equally unimpressed. The chief criticism is that one of the studies involved patients with heart failure, meaning the results aren't relevant to the general population. Participants also only reduced their sodium intake by fairly moderate increments, and were followed for relatively short periods, again, not enough to see a significant difference in their long-term health. To further lessen the credibility of the study, the editor-in-chief of the *Journal of Hypertension*,

Michael Alderman who accepted the paper, once worked as a consultant for the Salt Institute. As you might suspect, this Virginia-based advocacy group touts the benefits of higher sodium consumption while warning efforts to cut salt could be disastrous for the population's wellbeing.

Indeed the Salt Institute couldn't be more delighted with the recent research, as well as Campbell's announcement of its intention to up salt levels. "The scientific evidence is over-whelming," said Lori Roman, President of the Institute, clearly unconvinced of the criticism lobbed at the pro-sodium studies. "[I]t is time for the government to cease its costly and wasteful efforts to reduce salt consumption until it can conclusively prove a tangible benefit for all consumers."

But before you throw caution to the wind, and open up that bag of salt and vinegar chips in anticipation of Campbell's tastier potages, you might want to consider another study that was also published last week, this time in the *Archives of Internal Medicine*. Researchers from the Centers of Disease Prevention and Control concluded that Americans who consume a diet high in sodium and low in potassium have a 50% increased risk of death from any cause, and have twice the risk of death from heart attacks. The group found that high salt intake was associated with a 20% increased risk of death, while high potassium intake was associated with a 20% decreased risk of dying. Also, don't forget the link between a salt-heavy diet and high blood pressure is relatively well established, even the Cochrane Review couldn't undermine this widely accepted relationship.

So where does this leave Campbell's? In light of the lack of conclusive evidence linking sodium to an increased risk of cardiovascular disease, is the company justified in increasing salt? Perhaps the assertion that customers should have the right to choose whether they consume higher or lower levels of salt is in fact a fair and balanced one? After all, Campbell's still plans to include a number of low-sodium options among its soup offerings. And let's face an unfortunate reality; consumers are less concerned about salt in their diet than they are about other nutritional no-nos such as fat and sugar. The bottom line is that fat and sugar makes us well, fat, and there's no escaping this truth. We read it in magazines; we see it on TV, and even posters on the subway shout about the blubberizing impact of sugary, fatty foods. Salt, on the other hand, doesn't affect our appearance in the same way – although admittedly, it can lead to bloating and water retention, but not everyone is cognizant of this. So while we might compromise on taste to save our figures, we don't make the same allowances to save our *insides*. Indeed, Campbell's incoming CEO Denise Morrison was explicit in her analysis that sodium reduction is not a priority USP for many consumers.

Campbell's big mistake might have been boasting about its salt reduction initiatives. Change doesn't always sell. Remember when Coca-Cola launched New Coke in 1985, and accompanied the re-jigged recipe with a massive marketing campaign? The altered drink was a huge failure and the original formula had to be reinstated.

Who knows, had Coca-Cola kept the change quiet maybe we'd all be drinking New Coke now. Similarly, had Campbell's gone about reducing salt in small increments and not made a lot of noise about it, maybe its consumer base wouldn't have even noticed.

Unilever found in a 2007 study in the Netherlands that when consumers were given two identical samples of Lipton Cup-a-Soup and were told one had 25% less sodium, the majority of respondents said the soup labeled as low-salt tasted inferior.

Writer Nadia Arumugan raises some interesting points. As CKD patients, does it behoove us to keep our sodium levels low? I say it does, since hypertension plays a part in our disease. You need to remember that we are NOT part of the general population anymore. As I explained in **What Is It and How Did I Get It? Early Stage Chronic Kidney Disease**, CKD affects all your other medical issues.

It's Not Just Us

8/12/11   There's a chapter in **What Is It and How Did I Get It? Early Stage Chronic Kidney Disease** entitled, "Other Medical Issues While a CKD Patient." One of the items discussed in this chapter is medication and how it interacts with the kidneys. I keep harping about reading the labels of any medications you might need to take. Not only do you need to know what's in the medication and how it may interact with other medications you may be taking, but you need to know if the dosage prescribed has been changed, if there's a change in the formulation, and – most importantly – if this medication may be a danger to Chronic Kidney Disease patients.

Now it turns out that we are not the only ones who need to be so careful. Mary Brophy Marcus's article on USAToday.com has some interesting information for all of us.

Read the drug labels, avoid dangerous side effects

When Johnson & Johnson announced plans last week to lower the maximum dose for Extra Strength Tylenol, the news made some people rethink how often they take the drug and other over-the-counter medicines.

In an effort to reduce the risk of liver damage resulting from over-use of acetaminophen — the active ingredient in Tylenol — the drugmaker's McNeil division will soon cap the product's daily dose recommendation at 3,000 milligrams (a total of six 500-milligram pills a day) instead of the current 4,000 (eight pills a day).

Some experts say they also worry about overuse of other medications that consumers can purchase off pharmacy shelves without a prescription, such as the pain reliever ibuprofen, Theraflu for colds, and the antihistamine Benadryl.

"It's important for the public to realize all drugs have side effects. It doesn't matter if they're prescription, over-the-counter, herbals or nutritional supplements. If they have active ingredients, they have side effects and can interfere with normal body functions," says Brian Strom, director of the Center for Clinical Epidemiology and Biostatistics at the Perelman School of Medicine at the University of Pennsylvania.

He says Tylenol is an "extraordinarily" safe drug at proper doses, even though its overuse is a leading cause for liver transplants in patients with acute liver failure. But, he says, "It has a narrow therapeutic ratio. The toxic dose and the therapeutic dose are very close."

Other drugs also contain acetaminophen, such as over-the-counter cold remedies (Nyquil, Dayquil) and prescription Percocet and Vicodin. But many people aren't aware of this, and it can lead to overdoses. "People don't really read labels," Strom says. Changing the daily dose recommendation "was a good move, but it was not enough." He says manufacturers need to make it harder to overdo it with over-the-counter drugs that pose greater overdose risks, for example by packing drugs such as Tylenol in smaller quantities and doing away with "extra-strength" versions.

Other common, and commonly overused, over-the-counter drugs that concern experts include nonsteroidal anti-inflammatories (NSAIDS) such as naproxen (Aleve) and ibuprofen (Advil and Motrin), says Winston Parris, professor of anesthesiology and division chief for Pain Management at Duke University Medical Center.

 "You can have GI (gastrointestinal) problems, especially if you have a history of ulcers and bleeding," Parris says.

Overdosing on NSAIDs also can damage kidneys, says transplant pharmacist Lisa McDevitt, a clinical specialist in organ transplantation at Tufts Medical Center.

"We've seen patients come for kidney transplants who ended up with renal failure because of daily around-the-clock use of naproxen. It's not as common as Tylenol toxicity, though," she says. [This deals specifically with CKD patients like us.]

Overdoing it on Benadryl, used for allergies, is not uncommon either, says Sarah Anderson, an assistant professor of clinical pharmacy at the University of Colorado School of Pharmacy.

Though it won't cause organ failure in amounts higher than the daily recommended dose, Anderson says, "The big danger is its sedating side effects. That's dangerous from a driving standpoint or certain lines of work where heavy machinery is used, for example."

"People play loose and free with Benadryl," says Ausim Azizi, chair of the department of neurology at Temple University School of Medicine. "There are a lot of side effects. One is loss of memory in the immediate period after taking it, and disorientation in older people," he says.

Overuse can also cause serious drying side effects, especially in some with other health issues, says Anderson. "People with glaucoma and urinary retention, and men with prostate issues, can have more problems," she says.

Anderson says over-the-counter herbals stocked in drugstores are of concern, too, especially what she calls the "G" herbals. Ginkgo biloba and garlic supplements can put a person at risk for increased bleeding, she says, and many people don't realize the herbal drug Saint-John's-wort, used by some to self-treat depression, can decrease the effectiveness of oral contraceptives.

"Herbals are troublesome — there's no quality control," says Strom. "If we're lucky, they're placebos."

If you have a medical condition or you're on other drugs, Anderson says, you need to be vigilant. "Read labels and check things out with your physician and pharmacist," she says.

"All drugs do harm," says Strom. "We've decided for some, though, the toxicity is worth it."

Commonly used over-the-counter medications may carry risks, say experts.
Acetaminophen (Extra Strength Tylenol). For headaches, joint and muscle pain, fever.

Overuse risks: Liver damage or failure. May cause liver problems at lower doses in alcohol users, or in those who take other drugs containing acetaminophen.

Ibuprofen (Advil, Motrin), a nonsteroidal anti-inflammatory drug (NSAID). Reduces pain and swelling related to arthritis. Relieves headache, fever, menstrual cramps.

Overuse risks: Gastrointestinal pain, bleeding, Kidney damage.

Diphenhydramine (Benadryl), antihistamine used to prevent, reduce hay fever and other allergy symptoms.

Overuse risks: Memory loss and disorientation, especially in elderly. Drowsiness, dryness.

Loratadine (Claritin), antihistamine used to relieve hay fever, other allergy symptoms.

Overuse risks: Sleepiness, fast heart rate. May lose effectiveness over time. Claritin-D includes an additional active ingredient, pseudoephedrine sulfate, which may cause insomnia or restless-ness. Pseudoephedrine should not be taken with certain medications for Parkinsons, depression, psychiatric or other emotional conditions.

Dextromethorphan, a cough suppressant, and Doxylamine succinate, and antihistamine (NyQuil Cough).

Overuse risks: Can cause drowsiness, especially when mixed with sleeping medications and alcohol. Not to be taken with certain medications for Parkinsons, depression, psychiatric or other emotional conditions.

Ranitidine (Zantac), an acid reducer, treats ulcers and gastroesophageal reflux disease (GERD).

Overuse risks: May lose effectiveness over time. Long-term acid suppressor use could lead to poor absorption of some forms of calcium.

Okay, so it's annoying and the print on the package is small, but take the time to read it. It's another way to prolong your life.

A Simple Dip Stick Urine Test?

8/22/11   Those of you on Facebook [Why not like **SlowItDownCKD** on Facebook now that I've brought it up?] probably already know why last week's blogs weren't posted. Considering all the extra work for radio shows, book talks and public relations the book has produced, I'll be cutting down the blogs to once a week – on Monday.

Today's article is a bit technical, but basically it explains how a simple, non-invasive test can detect Chronic Kidney Disease. It's as easy as urinating into a cup and allowing your doctor to place a dip stick in your urine sample. You know I'm not a doctor, but I sincerely feel that if I'd been diagnosed earlier, I might have been able to do more to preserve more of my kidney function. I'm excited that this is becoming such a simple process.

Simple Urine Test Detects Silent Kidney Disease

Washington, DC — July 29, 2011 — A simple and inexpensive urine test routinely done in family doctors' offices may be the key to identifying individuals who are silently undergoing rapid kidney function decline, according to a study appearing in an upcoming issue of the *Journal of the American Society Nephrology* (JASN). Using this test could lead to potentially earlier and more effective treatments, lowering patients' risks for renal failure and premature death.

Approximately 60 million people globally have Chronic Kidney Disease. Early detection and prevention of kidney disease is the only way to prevent renal failure, but individuals with kidney disease often do not experience symptoms until later stages of the disease. Serial monitoring of kidney function in the general population would likely catch such silently progressing kidney disease early, but it would be too expensive.

William Clark, MD, The University of Western Ontario and London Health Sciences Centre, both in London, and Ontario, Canada, and his colleagues evaluated whether simple and routine screening tests for urine protein could be used to identify individuals at highest risk of rapid kidney function decline. These patients would benefit the most from serial kidney function monitoring and early treatments to prevent kidney failure.

The investigators followed 2,574 participants in a community-based clinic for an average of 7 years. They found that a positive dipstick urine test (a protein concentration of $>=1g/L$) was a strong predictor of rapid kidney function decline. Overall, 2.5% of participants in the study had a urinary protein concentration of $>=1g/L$ at the start of the study. If all of them were followed with serial monitoring of kidney function, one case of rapid kidney function decline would be identified for every 2.6 patients who were followed.

The test correctly identified whether or not individuals had rapid kidney function decline in 90.8% of participants, mislabeled 1.5% as having the condition, and missed 7.7% who were later identified as having the condition. Among those with certain risk factors, such as cardiovascular disease, age >60 years, diabetes, or hyper-tension, the probability of identifying rapid kidney function decline from serial kidney function measurements increased from 13% to 44% after incorporating a positive dipstick test.

"We showed that routine inexpensive urine dipstick screening in a population with and without risk factors will allow primary clinicians to follow fewer patients with serial monitoring to identify those with rapid kidney function decline that will potentially benefit from earlier referral and therapeutic intervention," said Dr. Clark.

This study was funded by peer-review grants from Kidney Foundation of Canada and the Ontario Ministry of Health.

Yes! Yes! Yes!

8/29/11   I read this *New York Times* article and jumped up ex-claiming, "He understands! He really understands!" The he to whom I referred is Dr. Joseph Vassalotti of Mount Sinai Medical Center and private practice in New York. He also just happens to be chief medical officer of the National Kidney Foundation.

If you read this blog, you know I wrote **What Is It and How Did I Get It? Early Stage Chronic Kidney Disease** because I didn't want anyone else to be in the position I'd been in: newly diag-nosed, scared, not taking in what my nephrologist was telling me, and not knowing that I could take a more active part in main-taining my kidney function nor how to do that. Dr. Vassalotti real-ized how new patients react to the information their doctors give them by simply asking a patient what he had heard. All the patient heard was the diagnose. But I'll let you read about this yourselves.

Doctors sharpen message on kidney disease
By JANE E. BRODY

Twenty-six million Americans have Chronic Kidney Disease, and avoiding complications depends heavily on how well patients care for themselves.

A patient with early stage kidney disease provided a recent wake-up call for Dr. Joseph Vassalotti, a leading kidney specialist. After explaining the diagnosis in great detail, the doctor asked his pa-tient to repeat what he had heard in his own words.

With a rather bored look on his face, the man said, "Kidney disease, yada yada yada yada."

Vassalotti, a nephrologist at Mount Sinai Medical Center in New York and chief medical officer of the National Kidney Foundation, was stunned. It was hardly the first time he had explained kidney disease to one of his patients, and he thought he knew how to help them recognize its seriousness and to motivate them to do what they could to forestall the day when their kidneys failed and dialysis or a transplant would be the only option for survival.

"I learned a lot from this patient," Vassalotti told me. "Clearly my explanation was not pitched correctly to fit his level of understanding and his attitude toward his health."

Twenty-six million Americans have Chronic Kidney Disease, which has a number of causes — most often diabetes and high blood pressure. As the kidneys begin to fail, the body's waste products build up in the bloodstream, leading to anemia, nerve damage, heart disease and other ailments.

As with heart disease and diabetes, avoiding these complications depends heavily on how well patients care for themselves. But the disease is symptomless, at least in the early stages, and many patients fail to appreciate that they are gradually heading toward a precipice.

The medical profession has been trying harder in recent years to communicate better with patients, but clearly there are serious impediments. Doctors are grappling with shortage of time and lack of training on how best to get needed information and advice across in terms that patients can hear and understand.

Too often, doctors speak in medicalese, a foreign language to their patients. Or they may be reluctant to place all the cards on the table, concerned that patients may become so fearful they fail to hear important information. Unlike Vassalotti, some doctors never ask patients what they understood.

Medicare now reimburses for educating patients with relatively advanced kidney disease, but not for those in the early stages.

MANY CARELESS PATIENTS

Communication is a two-way street, however, and patients with Chronic Kidney Disease also are contributing to its failure in several ways. Many lack health literacy. Unable to understand even simplified medical terms, they may misinterpret what a doctor tells them or forget it entirely.

They may be too intimidated to ask questions or request a clarification. They may regard all medical matters to be the doctor's purview. Or they may be fatalists who assume whatever will be, will be.

What kidney patients do, and don't do, can make a huge difference in the quality and length of their lives. Whether they follow through on medical advice depends heavily on what they know about their disease and what can make matters better or worse, Vassalotti said in an interview.

In a study published in March in *The American Journal of Kidney Disease*, a research team at Vanderbilt University Medical Center in Nashville uncovered serious knowledge gaps among 401 patients with various stages of the disease.

The team, headed by Dr. Kerri L. Cavanaugh, a nephrologist, pointed out that within the general population, most people with kidney disease don't know they have it. And among those who do know, a previous study of 676 patients with moderate to advanced kidney disease had found that more than a third knew little or nothing about it and nearly half knew nothing about treatment options should their kidneys fail completely.

Participants in the Vanderbilt study were being treated at the university's nephrology clinic for Chronic Kidney Disease. They ranged in age from 46 to 68; 53 percent were men, 83 percent were white and 94 percent had completed high school or higher. More than half had seen a nephrologist at least three times in the past year, and 17 percent had attended a kidney education session.

When asked whether they had Chronic Kidney Disease, however, more than a third answered "no." The 28-question survey revealed that only about 1 in 5 knew that protein in the urine was a sign of poor kidney function and that kidney disease often progresses without causing any symptoms.

Only 2 in 5 knew that controlling blood sugar is important in kidney disease, although more than 90 percent knew it is important to control blood pressure.

The usual lack of symptoms as kidney disease progresses is especially critical for patients to understand, because many fail to seek medical care or follow medical recommendations when they feel well. Dr. Julie Anne Wright, an author of the Vanderbilt study, said that it "highlights the need for providers to ensure that communication is not only delivered but understood by all parties involved."

LIFE-ENHANCING FACTS

Here is what everyone with Chronic Kidney Disease and those at increased risk of developing it should know.

• There are four main risk factors for kidney disease: diabetes, high blood pressure, age over 60 and a family history of the disease. Anyone with these risk factors should have a test of kidney function at least once a year, Vassalotti said. Members of certain ethnic groups are also at higher than average risk: blacks, Hispanics, Pacific Islanders and Native Americans.

• Two simple, relatively inexpensive tests, easily done during a routine doctor visit, can detect declining kidney function: a blood test called eGFR (for estimated glomerular filtration rate, a measure of kidney function) and urine albumin, which shows whether the kidneys are spilling protein.

• Early detection can delay progression to kidney failure, when dialysis or transplant is the only option. Good control of blood sugar, blood pressure, cholesterol levels and body weight can delay the loss of kidney function. Not smoking and getting regular physical activity and sleep are also important.

• Certain drugs and dyes are toxic to the kidneys and should be avoided by people with kidney disease. The drugs include painkillers like acetaminophen, aspirin and ibuprofen; laxatives and antacids that contain magnesium and aluminum (Mylanta and Milk of Magnesia); ulcer drugs like Tagamet and Zantac; decongestants like Sudafed; enemas that contain phosphorus (Fleet); and Alka-Seltzer, which is high in salt. Contrast dyes used for certain tests, like angiograms and some MRIs, can also be harmful to kidney patients.

• When kidney disease progresses, patients can develop symptoms like changes in urination; swelling in the legs, ankles, feet, hands or face; fatigue; skin rashes and itching; a metallic taste in the mouth; nausea and vomiting; shortness of breath; feeling cold even when it is warm; dizziness and trouble concentrating; and back or leg pain. If any of these occur, they should be brought to a doctor's attention without delay.

I immediately e-mailed Dr. Vassalotti and Ms. Brody to thank them for making this common knowledge. I only wish there was enough money in my bank account to get a copy of ***What Is It and How Did I Get It? Early Stage Chronic Kidney Disease*** to every newly diagnosed Chronic Kidney Disease patient.

But That's What I've Been Saying

9/5/11 Now that I've been able to stay home for more than a few days in a row and actually organize some of the papers on my desk this Labor Day weekend, I've come to realize the AMA [American Medical Association] is starting to think the same way I do. That's not as grandiose a statement as you might think.

If you heard **The Wellness Authors Show**'s interview about *What Is It and How Did I Get It? Early Stage Chronic Kidney Disease*, you heard me explain at one point that I look for patterns in my medical results. I also believe there are patterns in the development of diseases. I mean simple, logical progressions in deteriorating health. Of course, it's the doctors and researchers who establish the veracity of these patterns, but even a layman [like me] can see them.

I discovered this article at privatemdlabs.com. I like that the article suggests that PATIENTS bring this possibility to the attention of their doctors.

Metabolic syndrome shown to increase risk of kidney problems

Individuals who suffer from metabolic syndrome may benefit from talking to their doctor about kidney testing, as new research shows that the condition significantly increases the risk of renal complications.

Metabolic syndrome is a collection of conditions that include unhealthy cholesterol, high blood pressure, insulin resistance and excess abdominal fat. It is known to increase a person's chances of developing heart disease and diabetes, but the new study is among the first to connect it to kidney risk.

For the study, researchers from the Cleveland Clinic analyzed the findings of 11 previously published studies involving more than

30,000 participants. The results showed that individuals with metabolic syndrome were 55 percent more likely to develop kidney problems. Low kidney function, which is an early sign of kidney disease, a condition that often leads to organ failure, was the most common problem.

The researchers said that primary care physicians should be aware of these findings and recommend kidney testing to their patients when appropriate. Counseling individuals with the condition on their risk of developing renal diseases could enable them to make lifestyle changes before severe harm is done to the organ.

One Third of the Three Ps

9/12/11 I've written about the three Ps and salt in ***What Is It and How Did I Get It? Early Stage Chronic Kidney Disease*** and in the blog, too. The one third of the three Ps discussed in this article from *The Los Angeles Times* is potassium. To refresh your memory, potassium counteracts sodium's effect on blood pressure.

There was a banana in my breakfast; that's one fruit unit on the renal diet and 467 mg of potassium. This is an example of just how easy it is to incorporate potassium into your meals.

In with potassium, out with sodium

People whose diets have roughly equal amounts of sodium and potassium are at the lowest risk of dying from heart attack and stroke, new study finds.

For decades now, we've heard that too much sodium can cause hypertension and raise the risk of cardiovascular disease. People have paid far less attention to potassium, a mineral that has opposite effects on health: Get enough of it, and it can actually lower your blood pressure and protect your heart.

Now a study of more than 12,000 adults has underscored something that doctors and nutritionists have been saying for years: If you watch your sodium but ignore potassium, you're missing an important part of the picture.

The study, published in the July 11 issue of the journal *Archives of Internal Medicine*, found that people whose diets had the lowest ratio of sodium to potassium (translating to roughly equal amounts of the two nutrients) were at the lowest risk of dying from heart attack and stroke. Those who consumed the highest amounts of sodium relative to potassium — 50% more, on average — had a 46% higher risk of dying from cardiovascular-related illness.

However, the study did not prove a cause-and-effect relationship, said coauthor Dr. Elena Kuklina, a nutritional epidemiologist at the U.S. Centers for Disease Control and Prevention in Atlanta. "We found some relationship between diet and mortality, but since it was not a clinical trial, we can't say for sure that diet is a cause of mortality." To show cause and effect, scientists would have to put people on set diets, randomly assigned, for a long period of time and follow them until they died — an inordinately difficult undertaking.

Though doctors know that potassium plays a significant role in heart health, many are reluctant to take any attention away from sodium, said Dr. Gordon Tomaselli, president of the American Heart Assn. and chief of cardiology at Johns Hopkins University in Baltimore. "Sodium is important," he reiterated. People can improve their cardiovascular health simply by eating less of it, he said, and any benefit from high potassium foods would be a bonus.

The new study followed 12,267 adults for an average of 14.8 years. Researchers used dietary surveys to estimate the potassium and sodium intakes at the start of the study. As expected, people who consumed the most sodium were also the most likely to die during the study — a 73% increase over those who consumed the least sodium — while people who consumed the most potassium had relatively low death rates — a 39% lower risk than those who consumed the least.

But the balance between sodium and potassium mattered, too. Those participants who got high sodium and low potassium had the highest death rates of all: a 46% higher risk of dying from any cause than those who ate equal proportions of the nutrients.

They were especially vulnerable to death from heart attack, for which the risks doubled.

Tomaselli said the study was noteworthy because of the large number of participants representing a cross-section of Americans and because they were followed for long enough to include a significant number of deaths. However, dietary intake was not directly measured but was estimated based on each subject's memory. And even assuming that the estimates are accurate, Tomaselli noted that diets heavy in sodium and light in potassium may be unhealthful in ways that have little to do directly with the two minerals.

A previous study, published in the *Archives of Internal Medicine* in 2009, also found an association between cardiovascular disease and the balance between sodium and potassium. Rather than estimating dietary intake, researchers measured actual levels of sodium and potassium in the urine of 2,275 subjects with prehypertension (diastolic blood pressure between 80 and 89) and followed them for 10 to 15 years.

Again, higher sodium seemed to increase the risk of heart attack and stroke, and potassium seemed to have the opposite effect. But the only association that passed muster statistically was the balance between sodium and potassium. "The size of the effect was very similar to the CDC study," noted study coauthor Nancy Cook, a researcher in preventative medicine at Brigham and Women's Hospital in Boston.

Focusing on the ratio between sodium and potassium makes biological sense because the minerals are known to have opposite effects on blood pressure, Kuklina said. Sodium generally increases blood pressure and signals the body to retain fluids. Potassium, however, relaxes blood vessels, lowers blood pressure and helps rid the body of excess fluids.

The U.S. dietary guidelines recommend limiting sodium intake to 2,300 milligrams per day and even lower — 1,500 mg — for those 51 and older and people of any age who are African American or have high blood pressure, kidney disease or diabetes. (The American Heart Assn. recently switched to a target of 1,500 mg per day for everyone.)

The average daily intake of sodium by Americans is much higher than that — more than 3,400 mg per day, according to CDC estimates. Recommended potassium intake is 4,700 mg per day, but average U.S. intake is in the range of only 2,000-2,500 mg per day, Cook said.

For those whose eyes already glaze over when told to read nutrition labels, there's a simpler way to reduce sodium and increase potassium in your diet: Choose fresh, whole foods over packaged, processed ones. More than 75% of American sodium intake comes in the form of processed foods, Kuklina said. And the best potassium sources are fruits and vegetables such as potatoes, bananas, grapes, carrots, greens and citrus fruits. Simply by eating fewer processed foods you can decrease your sodium intake and increase your potassium intake in one fell swoop.

"The message is to eat a healthy balanced diet," Kuklina said. "It's good for health in general and for cardiovascular health."

A Garden of Help

9/19/11   I was raised in a meat and potatoes eating family with a number of high blood pressure suffering members. Reading this article from *Renal & Urology News* got me to wondering... [especially since high blood pressure is considered one of the causes of Chronic Kidney Disease].

Fruits, Vegetables Boost BP Control

A diet rich in fruits and vegetables can lower blood pressure (BP) in patients with coronary heart disease (CHD), according to data presented at the European Society of Cardiology annual meeting.

The results also show that the mean fruit and vegetable intake needed to achieve target BP is about 580 grams per day. "The main take-away message is that an achievable, daily intake of fruit and vegetables has a significant beneficial effect on blood pressure, irrespective of health status, which has potentially huge implications for the population at large and overall public health," Vernon Heazlewood, MD, senior staff specialist at Caboolture Hospital Queensland Health in Caboolture , Australia, told *Renal & Urology News*. "The message is simple yet profound in its health impact."

Dr. Heazlewood and colleagues conducted a post-hoc analysis of the EUROACTION study, which tested the use of a preventive cardiology program addressing lifestyle and medical risk factor management in patients with

CHD and high-risk patients in eight European countries. Their analysis aimed primarily to determine if there was a relationship between fruit and vegetable consumption and blood pressure outcomes as continuous variables.

"The benefit of diet and lifestyle in assisting blood pressure control has been confirmed in prior studies but these trials have been performed in healthy individuals under strict conditions and in short time frames – usually from two to six months," Dr. Heazlewood pointed out. "Furthermore, none has assessed the impact of fruit and vegetable consumption alone nor examined the effect of a more realistic dietary fruit and vegetable target of five or more portions per day (for a total of more than 400 grams per day) in lieu of at least eight to nine portions a day."

The analysis included 942 patients younger than 80 years who had been hospitalized with acute coronary syndrome or angina.

The desirable BP target was 140/90 mm Hg (or 130/85 mm Hg in individuals with diabetes) and the fruit and vegetable target was 400 grams or more per day. Participants were urged to increase their intake of oily fish, limit their alcohol intake, and exercise regularly.

Results showed that higher daily fruit and vegetable consumption was associated with lower diastolic and systolic pressures.

The mean daily fruit and vegetable consumption in those patients achieving the BP target was 583 grams compared with 536 grams in those individuals not reaching their BP target, for a mean difference of 47 grams per day.

In patients with uncontrolled systolic pressure (defined as a pressure of 140 mm Hg or higher), the mean daily fruit and vegetable intake was 541 grams compared with 577 grams in individuals those with systolic pressure below 140 mm Hg, for a mean difference of 36 grams per day.

Similarly for uncontrolled diastolic pressure (defined as a diastolic pressure higher than 90 mm Hg), the mean daily fruit and vegetable intake was 485 grams compared with 576 grams with controlled diastolic pressure, for a mean difference of 91 grams.

Additionally, the results showed that individual study sites where a fruit and vegetable target consumption was achieved were more likely to reach blood pressure targets.

Dr. Heazlewood emphasized that the fact that the study was a post-hoc analysis may represent a limitation. Also, validation and "regularity" of fruit and vegetable consumption as well as the extent of compliance with drug treatment were not known.

He added, however, that the findings supporting an association of fruit and vegetable consumption on blood pressure outcomes are consistent with the literature showing similar findings in healthy individuals.

Why is High Blood Pressure Important Again?

9/26/11   Just as I found myself thinking it was time for a reminder of the importance of controlling high blood pressure since it plays such an intricate role in CKD, ScienceDaily ran this article.

Kidney damage and high blood pressure: faulty filtration allows detrimental enzymes to wreak havoc on fluid balance, research suggests

The kidney performs several vital functions. It filters blood, removes waste products from the body, balances the body's fluids, and releases hormones that regulate blood pressure. A number of diseases and conditions can damage the kidney's filtration apparatus, such as diabetes and immune disorders. This damage leads to a condition called nephrotic syndrome, which is characterized by protein in the urine, high cholesterol and triglycerides, and swelling (edema). People with nephrotic syndrome retain salt and water in their bodies and develop swelling and high blood pressure as a result.

Scientists have now begun to understand kidney damage on a cellular level and how the activity of certain molecules in damaged kidneys contributes to salt and water retention in nephrotic syndrome.

Faulty Filtration

The kidneys are marvels of filtration, processing roughly 150 to 200 quarts of blood each day through tiny structures called nephrons. There are about 1 million nephrons per kidney, and each nephron consists of a filtering unit of blood vessels called a glomerulus, which is attached to a tubule. Filtered blood enters the tubule, where various substances are either added to or removed from the filtrate as necessary, and most of the filtered sodium and water is removed. The filtrate that exits the tubule is excreted as urine.

In nephrotic syndrome, a damaged filtration barrier allows substances that are not normally filtered to appear in the filtrate. One of these substances is the protein plasminogen, which is converted in kidney tubules to the protease plasmin. In their research, Thomas R. Kleyman, Professor of Medicine and of Cell biology and Physiology at the University of Pittsburgh School of Medicine and the Symposium's co-organizer, and Ole Skøtt, Professor of Physiology and Pharmacology and Dean at the University of Southern Denmark in Odense, independently found that plasmin plays a role in activating the epithelial sodium channel (ENaC) on cells in the nephron. ENaC is a protein embedded in cell membranes that facilitates the absorption of filtered sodium from tubules. When ENaC becomes overactive, excessive absorption of filtered sodium may lead to sodium and water retention.

According to Dr. Kleyman, these findings provide an explanation of how damage to the glomeruli in the kidney's nephrons leads to edema and high blood pressure. Dr. Kleyman explains: "When plasminogen is cleaved, it can act on several targets. One of those targets is ENaC. Another is the protein prostasin, which, once cleaved, will activate ENaC, as well."

Dr. Kleyman noted the implications these findings have for treating edema and high blood pressure in patients suffering from nephrotic syndrome. "This is important because if plasmin activates ENaC, it suggests that targeting ENaC in the kidneys with ENaC inhibitors may be a treatment option."

While CKD and Nephrotic Syndrome are not the same, the explanation of the inter-relationship between high blood pressure and kidney damage is very clear in this article.

There Goes Another Reason To Enjoy Carbs – Kapop

10/3/11   Milk and soy protein supplements may be better than carb supplements for lowering systolic blood pressure

Strike another blow for refined carbs: A study released today finds that soy and milk protein supplements may be associated with lower blood pressure more than refined carbohydrate supplements.

The study, published online in *Circulation: Journal of the American Heart Assn.*, put 352 adults who were at risk for high blood pressure or who had mild hypertension on various rounds of supplements. The participants were given 40 grams of powdered soy, milk or refined complex carb supplements daily for eight weeks, and had their blood pressure taken at various intervals during the trial. They were told to keep their calories the same, as well as their usual sodium consumption and amount they exercised.

Although none of the groups experienced a significant drop in diastolic blood pressure readings, there were differences in systolic readings. A systolic reading (the top number) measures the force put on the arteries when the heart contracts, pushing blood through the arteries. A diastolic reading (the bottom number) measures the force in the arteries between heart beats. Those who took the milk protein supplement had an average 2.3-mmHg lower systolic blood pressure compared with when they had the carb supplement. And those who had the soy protein supplement saw an average 2-mmHg drop in systolic pressure compared with the carb supplement.

Blood pressure readings didn't change substantially during the time the study participants took the carb supplement.

"Some previous observational research on eating carbohydrates inconsistently suggested that a high carbohydrate diet might help reduce blood pressure," said the study's lead author, Dr. Jiang He, in a news release. He, an epidemiologist at Tulane University School of Public Health and Tropical Medicine in New Orleans, added, "In contrast, our clinical trial directly compares soy protein with milk protein on blood pressure, and shows they both lower blood pressure better than carbohydrates."

As the grand-daughter of a Ukrainian miller, I have always loved bread. When other children had candy or cookies and milk as a snack, in my childhood home we had great slabs of rye, pumpernickel or corn bread sliced from an enormous wheel and then slathered with chicken fat for the adults [No comment.] or butter [Well, that's a little better.]. It was heavenly, so I continued my love of bread into adulthood but never graduated to the adult's chicken fat, preferring to stick to butter, then margarine when that was claimed to be healthier and back to butter since I've been diagnosed with Chronic Kidney Disease.

When life got hard, I relied on my comfort food secure in the knowledge that, although I was adding calories, I was helping to lower my blood pressure. That same blood pressure that the hard times were causing to rise... and rise... and rise.

And now this! My first – albeit slightly irreverent – reaction to this article was, "Is nothing sacred anymore!!!!" screamed in anguish. I wanted my bread. Re-reading the article I see I can have it – keeping within the six carbohydrate units on my renal diet, naturally – but it just might not be helping to lower my blood pressure. Considering I only have four ounces of dairy on this same diet, I'm just not sure how much this information will be of use to me. You, however, may have much more use for this interesting, if slightly unsettling, information.

A Bunch of Reasons to Weight Train

10/10/11   One of my bailiwicks is finding reasons to exercise. I love to dance, but not the half hour drive there and then the one back from the swing dance clubs – so I don't go as often as I'd like to. Walking tapes are fun; I start smiling ten minutes in, but they can become redundant. I rely on the indoor exercise bike quite a lot in the extreme heat out here. I still race around the big box stores, too, and bowl whenever the opportunity presents itself. Every once in a while, I'll go to an aerobics class at the local community center or the college.

But it seemed to me that most of my exercising dealt with the lower half of my body. What about the rest of me, I wondered. That's when I started surfing the internet and came up with the following article. Hmmm, I have weights right here in the house….

Strength training does more than bulk up muscles. It may reduce depression, give older people better cognitive function, boost good cholesterol and more.

Strength training has strong-armed its way beyond the realm of bodybuilding. A growing body of research shows that working out with weights has health benefits beyond simply bulking up one's muscles and strengthening bones. Studies are finding that more lean muscle mass may allow kidney dialysis patients to live longer, give older people better cognitive function, reduce depression, boost good cholesterol, lessen the swelling and discomfort of lymphedema after breast cancer and help lower the risk of diabetes.

"Muscle is our largest metabolically active organ, and that's the backdrop that people usually forget," said Kent Adams, director of the exercise physiology lab at Cal State Monterey Bay. Strengthening the muscles "has a ripple effect throughout the body on things like metabolic syndrome and obesity."

Historically, strength training was limited to athletes, but in the last 20 years, its popularity has spread to the general public, said Jeffrey Potteiger, an exercise physiologist at Grand Valley State University in Grand Rapids, Mich., and a fellow of the American College of Sports Medicine. "One can argue that if you don't do some resistance training through your lifespan, you're missing out on some benefits, especially as you get older or battle weight gain," he said.

When we hit middle age, muscle mass gradually diminishes by up to about 1% a year in a process called sarcopenia. Women also are in danger of losing bone mass as they age, especially after the onset of menopause. Some studies have shown that moderate to intense strength training not only builds skeletal muscle but increases bone density as well.

Strength training often takes a back seat to cardiovascular training, but it can benefit the heart in ways that its more popular cousin can't. During cardio exercise, the heart loads up with blood and pumps it out to the rest of the body: As a result, Potteiger said, "the heart gets better and more efficient at pumping."

But during resistance training, muscles generate more force than they do during endurance exercises, and the heart is no exception, Potteiger said. During a strength workout, the heart's muscle tissue contracts forcefully to push the blood out. Like all muscles, stress causes small tears in the muscle fibers. When the body repairs those tears, muscles grow. The result is a stronger heart, not just one that's more efficient at pumping.

Another big advantage of working out with weights is improving glucose metabolism, which can reduce the risk of diabetes. Strength training boosts the number of proteins that take glucose out of the blood and transport it into the skeletal muscle, giving the muscles more energy and lowering overall blood-glucose levels.

"If you have uncontrolled glucose levels," Potteiger said, "that can lead to kidney damage, damage to the circulatory system and loss of eyesight."

The benefits don't end there. A 2010 study in the *Clinical Journal of the American Society of Nephrology* suggested that people on dialysis can benefit from building muscle. Researchers found that kidney dialysis patients who had the most lean muscle mass — a measurement derived from the circumference of the mid-arm muscle — were 37% less likely to die than the patients who had the least.

"This is something that has an impact on survival," said Dr. Kamyar Kalantar-Zadeh, a principal researcher at the Los Angeles Biomedical Research Institute and coauthor of the study. "It's not just about having more muscle and looking better — we're talking about life and death."

Even people who already have Chronic Kidney Disease could benefit from strength workouts. Germany began to incorporate modified exercise equipment into dialysis treatment centers in 1995, and a 2004 study in the *American Journal of Kidney Diseases* examining that policy found that exercise may improve the efficiency of dialysis by increasing blood flow through the muscle and improving phosphate removal.

The brain may get a boost from the body's extra muscle as well. A 2010 study in *Archives of Internal Medicine* found that women ages 65 to 75 who did resistance training sessions once or twice a week over the course of a year improved their cognitive performance, while those who focused on balance and tone training declined slightly. One reason for the improvement, researchers believe, may be that strength training triggers the production of a protein beneficial for brain growth.

This study was triggered by another that looked at resistance training as a way to reduce the risk of falls in older people, said coauthor Teresa Liu-Ambrose, a researcher at the University of British Columbia's Centre for Hip Health and Mobility in Vancouver. As the study progressed, she said she noticed that participants "were able to take on new tasks, like taking the bus by themselves. They were able to prepare and plan for things and execute them."

Strength training could be easier for people with mobility problems who might find it easier to navigate a stationary weight than a moving treadmill.

"It's never too late to start," Adams said. "The benefits are great."

Did you notice the mention of glucose levels? While my own doctor has never mentioned them to me, other nephrologists and hospital renal department chiefs have. They're important. Start paying attention to them.

Jab or Shot: The Message Is the Same

10/17/11   As I dutifully sat in my local CVS Minute Clinic receiving a flu shot, I concentrated on two things: the chatter my pharmacist so thoughtfully provided to distract me from the actual injection and why I was doing this. Once back home, I caste around on the internet for some kind of cogent explanation and stumbled upon this article from England's Department of Health. I've only provided the relevant parts of the article. A couple of notes before you start reading: unfortunately, the vaccination is not free here in the states [The UK has socialized medical care.] and the English call a shot 'a jab.'

Seasonal flu occurs every year, usually in the winter. It's a highly infectious disease caused by a number of flu viruses. The most likely viruses that will cause flu each year are identified in advance and vaccines are then produced to closely match them. As with most seasonal flu vaccines, this year's vaccine will protect against three types of flu virus.

Isn't flu just a heavy cold?

No. Colds are much less serious and usually start gradually with a stuffy or runny nose and a sore throat.

How do I know when I've got flu?

Flu symptoms hit you suddenly and sometimes severely. They usually include fever, chills, headaches and aching muscles, and you can often get a cough and sore throat at the same time. Flu is caused by viruses and not bacteria, so antibiotics won't treat it.

What harm can seasonal flu do?

People sometimes think a bad cold is flu, but having flu can be much worse than a cold and you may need to stay in bed for a few days if you have flu. Some people are more susceptible to the effects of seasonal flu. For them it can increase the risk of developing more serious illnesses such as bronchitis and pneumonia, or can make existing conditions worse. In the worst cases, seasonal flu can result in a stay in hospital, or even death.

Am I at greater risk from the effects of seasonal flu?

Even if you feel healthy, you should definitely consider having the free seasonal flu vaccination if you have:
- a heart problem
- a chest complaint or breathing difficulties, including bronchitis or emphysema
- ***a kidney disease* [I bolded and italicized this for obvious reasons.]**
- lowered immunity due to disease or treatment (such as steroid medication or cancer treatment)
- a liver disease
- had a stroke or a transient ischemic attack (TIA)
- diabetes
- a neurological condition, for example multiple sclerosis (MS) or cerebral palsy
- a problem with your spleen, for example sickle cell disease, or you have had your spleen removed.

Don't wait until there is a flu outbreak this winter: contact your GP or practice nurse now to get your seasonal flu jab.

From Pot to Potassium

10/24/11   As a child of the 60s, I encountered pot [marijuana] everywhere I went. I was a college student and went wherever college students went. The difference between my peers and me is that I was so naive I didn't recognize what I was smelling. My folks were far savvier about this topic than I was since my mother routinely checked my eyes whenever I came home from socializing. I didn't know what she was looking for, but she did.

Then, as we all did, I grew up. I finished college, started teaching, got married, had children, bought a house, got divorced and developed Chronic Kidney Disease. That's where the potassium comes in. You know we [as Chronic Kidney Disease sufferers] have to limit the amount of potassium we ingest.

Medline delivered this incredibly informative article to my inbox this week. It is written so well and in such a manner that even the most stunned of the newly diagnosed can understand it that I've reproduced most of it here.

INTRODUCTION

Potassium is a mineral that is found in many foods. It keeps the heart beating regularly, helps to maintain fluid balance, and allows the nerves and muscles to work properly.

The kidneys maintain the correct level of potassium in the blood. People who take certain medicines or who have Chronic Kidney Disease must limit the amount of potassium in their diet to keep their potassium level close to normal.

WHY SHOULD I REDUCE POTASSIUM IN MY DIET?

Normally, the level of potassium in your body is balanced by eating foods that contain potassium and getting rid of excess potassium in the urine. However, some people with Chronic Kidney Disease cannot get rid of enough potassium in their urine because the kidneys do not work well.

In these people, the level of potassium in the blood can become higher than normal, causing a condition known as hyperkalemia (hyper=high, kal=potassium, emia=in the blood). Eating a low potassium diet can lower the risk of developing hyperkalemia.

The potassium level is measured by taking a small sample of blood from a vein. A typical normal range for potassium is 3.5 to 5 meq/L. A level greater than 6 meq/L is considered dangerous. A low level can be dangerous as well.

Hyperkalemia does not usually cause noticeable symptoms until the potassium level is very high. At this level, dangerous complications can develop, including an irregular heart rhythm or severe muscle weakness or paralysis.

HOW MUCH POTASSIUM DO I NEED?

In general, experts recommend eating a diet that contains at least 4700 mg of potassium per day. However, most people with Chronic Kidney Disease should eat less than 1500 to 2700 mg of potassium per day. A registered dietitian or nutritionist [The government pays for you to see the nutritionist attached to your nephrologist's practice.] can help to create a low potassium meal plan. An example of one such plan includes:

- Fruit — One to three servings of low-potassium fruit per day
- Vegetables — Two to three servings of low-potassium vegetables per day
- Dairy and calcium rich foods — One to two servings of low-potassium choices per day

- Meat and meat alternatives — Three to seven servings of low-potassium choices per day (approximately 15 percent of calories)
- Grains — Four to seven servings of low-potassium grains per day

[Does this remind you of your CKD diet? It should.]

HOW DO I CUT DOWN ON POTASSIUM?

- Almost all foods contain some potassium, so the key is to choose foods with a low potassium level, when possible.
- Notice the serving size when calculating the amount of potassium in a food; a large serving of a low potassium food may have more potassium than a small serving of a food with a high level of potassium.
- Drain canned vegetables, fruits, and meats before serving.

A process of "leaching" can reduce the amount of potassium in some vegetables. You can eat low potassium foods regularly, but watch your portion size since potassium can quickly add up if you eat a large portion.

Reducing potassium levels in vegetables — It is possible to remove some of the potassium in certain vegetables with high potassium levels. Leaching is a process of soaking raw or frozen vegetables in water for at least two hours before cooking to "pull" some of the potassium out of the food and into the water. You should not eat these vegetables frequently because there is still a lot of potassium in the food after leaching.

- Wash and then cut the raw vegetable into thin slices. Vegetables with a skin (eg, potatoes, carrots, beets, rutabagas) should be peeled before slicing.
- Rinse the cut vegetables in warm water.

- Soak the vegetables for at least two hours or overnight. Use a large amount of unsalted warm water (approximately 10 parts water to 1 part vegetables). If possible, change the water every four hours. Drain the soaking water.
- Rinse the vegetables again with warm water.
- Cook vegetables as desired, using a large amount of unsalted water (approximately 5 parts water to 1 part vegetables).
- Drain the cooking water.

[You can find samples of low and high potassium menus online. The information in this blog is from UpToDate.com. There are also phone apps available to count potassium.]

Foods with high levels of potassium

Grains
Whole-grain breads, wheat bran, granola and granola bars

Beverages
Sports drinks (Gatorade, etc.), instant breakfast mix, soy milk

Snack foods
Peanut butter (2 tablespoons), nuts or seeds (1 ounce), fig cookies, chocolate (1.5 to 2 ounces), molasses (1 tablespoon)

Fruits
Apricots, avocado (¼ whole), bananas (½ whole), coconut, melon (cantaloupe and honeydew), kiwi, mango, nectarines, oranges, orange juice, papaya, pears (fresh), plantains, pomegranate (and juice), dried fruits (apricots (5 halves), dates (5), figs, prunes, raisins), prune juice, yams

Vegetables
Bamboo shoots, baked or refried beans, beets, broccoli (cooked), Brussels sprouts, cabbage (raw), carrots (raw), chard, greens (except kale), kohlrabi, olives, mushrooms (canned), potatoes (white and sweet), parsnips, pickles, pumpkin, rutabaga, sauerkraut, spinach (cooked), squash (acorn, butternut, hubbard), tomato, tomato sauce, tomato juice, and vegetable juice cocktail

Dairy products
Milk and milk products, buttermilk, yogurt

Proteins
(3-ounce serving) Clams, sardines, scallops, lobster, whitefish, salmon (and most other fish), ground beef, sirloin steak (and most other beef products), pinto beans, kidney beans, black beans, navy beans (and most other peas and beans, serving size is ½ cup)

Soups
Salt-free soups and low-sodium bouillon cubes, unsalted broth

Condiments
Imitation bacon bits, lite salt or salt substitutes (avoid completely)

Unless noted, one serving is ½ cup (4 ounces). These foods have greater than 250 mg of potassium per serving and should be avoided or eaten in very small portions if you have been told to eat a low-potassium diet.

Reducing potassium levels in vegetables —Foods with low levels of Potassium

Grains
Foods prepared with white flour (eg, pasta, bread), white rice

Beverages
Non-dairy creamer, fruit punch, drink mixes (eg, Kool-Aid), tea (<2 cups or 16 ounces per day), coffee (<1 cup or 8 ounces per day)

Sweets
Angel or yellow cake, pies without chocolate or high-potassium fruit, cookies without nuts or chocolate

Fruits
Apples (1), apple juice, applesauce, apricots (canned), blackberries, blueberries, cherries, cranberries, fruit cocktail (drained), grapes, grape juice, grapefruit (½), mandarin oranges, peaches (½ fresh or ½ cup canned), pears (1 small fresh or ½ cup canned), pineapple and juice, plums (1 whole), raspberries, strawberries, tangerine (1 whole), watermelon (1 cup)

Vegetables
Alfalfa sprouts, asparagus (6 spears), green or wax beans, cabbage (cooked), carrots (cooked), cauliflower, celery (1 stalk), corn (½ fresh ear or ½ cup), cucumber, eggplant, kale, lettuce, mushrooms (fresh), okra, onions, parsley, green peas, green peppers, radish, rhubarb, water chestnuts (canned, drained), watercress, spinach (raw, 1 cup), squash (yellow), zucchini

Proteins
Chicken, turkey (3 ounces), tuna, eggs, baloney, shrimp, sunflower or pumpkin seeds (1 ounce), raw walnuts, almonds, cashews, or peanuts (all 1 ounce), flax seeds (2 tablespoons ground), unsalted peanut butter (1 tablespoon)

Dairy products
Cheddar or swiss cheese (1 ounce), cottage cheese (½ cup)

Unless noted, one serving is ½ cup (4 ounces). These foods have a low level of potassium (less than 250 mg potassium per serving on average).

You can eat these low potassium foods, but be sure to watch your portion size since potassium can quickly add up if you eat a large portion.

Too Comfortable?

10/31/11 I had today's blog practically completed in my mind when I ran across this essay on The New York Times.com. I've repeatedly argued that you have to be able to talk to your nephrologist and dietitian. I'm always questioning if I can be comfortable with my own doctors, but maybe I'm placing too much emphasis on this. I have a strong belief that things happen for a reason, even if we don't know what that reason is. Is that why this essay popped up just as I was starting today's blog? Read it and decide for yourself.

Downside of Doctors Who Feel Your Pain

When I started my medical internship, my father the doctor told me that, when he was an intern, the competence of his colleagues was inversely proportional to how much their patients liked them. My heart sank. I had the likability market covered.

You wanted eye contact? I could give you eye contact. You wanted someone to nod and say, "I understand your pain"? Empathy may as well have been my middle name. But actually tending to the acute medical issues of sick patients in the middle of the night? Interpersonal skills alone were not going to cut it. Medicine, like education, business and fashion, is subject to fads. Hormone replacement therapy. Radical mastectomy. Bloodletting. The latest? Breeding nice doctors. It's all the rage.

A wealthy Chicago couple recently donated $42 million to the University of Chicago Medical Center for the creation of an institute to improve the doctor-patient relationship. Already many medical schools are changing their admissions process to weed out candidates who communicate poorly. And now, to become licensed physicians, medical students must pass a "clinical skills" exam assessing, among other proficiencies, how well they acknowledge patient concerns, ask about feelings and show empathy.

The ideal physician surely possesses both competence and compassion. But will our quest to eradicate the coldhearted physician know-it-all be another fad with consequences we may later regret?

How do we even measure these skills? Those of us who have ever fallen in love with someone we once hated know that sincere empathy can take time to discover. During one of my clinical training sessions, a patient told me no physician had ever made her feel more at ease. The next cautioned that I made too much eye contact, sat too close and "invaded" her personal space. After briefly feeling like a sex offender, I realized the process, though well intentioned, was flawed.

Proponents of weeding out students who lack interpersonal skills argue that communication errors are at the root of medical mistakes. But we have no data to suggest that medical students who sit close but not too close make any fewer mistakes than their less-communicative colleagues. That awkward medical student in the corner who obsessively follows a checklist may make fewer procedural mistakes than his charming friend who lights up the room.

In fact, qualities suggestive of extroversion do not necessarily track with leadership or altruism. Adam Grant, an organizational psychologist at the Wharton School of the University of Pennsylvania, recently led several studies suggesting that extroverts, when grouped together, competed excessively and undermined one another's productivity. The introverts were better listeners and enhanced group performance. With the future of health care more uncertain than ever, do we want to be turning away these cooperative, albeit reticent minds?

I worry, finally, that this focus on interpersonal skills inevitably feeds our cost and quality crisis.

As a runner with serial overuse injuries, I am as guilty as anyone of conflating the most sympathetic doctor with the one who gives me what I want — for me, always an M.R.I. But in a culture that values novel technology above all else, undue emphasis on interpersonal skills may make it only more difficult for patients to discern good medicine from that which makes us feel most understood.

The beauty of clinical medicine is that we constantly question our latest wisdom. How we select and train medical students may be more difficult to evaluate than the effect of a vitamin supplement, but that does not excuse us from subjecting our novel approaches, including an emphasis on glad-handing patients, to the same investigative rigor.

I like to think my father was wrong about the relationship between clinical acumen and interpersonal skills. Regarding another piece of wisdom he shared, however, I'm certain he is right.

"Dad," I often asked as a child, "who is smarter, you or Mom?"

"Well, Lisa," he would answer, "there are different kinds of smart."

Glad to Know I'm Not the Only Optimist Out There

11/7/11   Sometimes people stop me when we're talking just to tell me they are impressed with my optimism in the face of my disease... and I'm dumbfounded. "Doesn't everyone with CKD keep living their lives?" I've wondered again and again when I hear this comment.

Then I remember a nephrologist who accused me of being so involved with my disease that he thought I would just give up and become a professional patient. He is obviously one of those doctors who just doesn't take the time to know his patients. But, more importantly, he's one that doesn't understand how important it is to make sure optimism is part of the treatment plan.

In searching CKD blogs, news reports and anything else I can find that relates to CKD each week, I stumbled upon this one and thrilled at its message. I am NOT the only optimist out there! While I don't necessarily agree with all this author espouses, there's enough here that makes me think the message is well worth the read.

At the top of their blog page they run the message: "**Live Now** is a movement to start living on your terms, with hope, optimism and strength." Their philosophy seems to be "Kidney disease doesn't define your life – you do. It's time to get up, get out and live for today." They'll get no argument from me.

Get That Flu Shot!

11/14/11   I've written in another blog about getting a flu shot. I also mentioned my pharmacist kindly chatting with me so I wouldn't be so uncomfortable with yet another puncture. I was already enduring these at least four, if not six, times a year for blood tests. I don't think I mentioned what he chatted about. He knew about the book and the blog, so we talked about how the flu affects CKD patients.

He told me a few things I didn't know and I told him a few he didn't know [Could have knocked me over with a feather when I realized I knew some information this intelligent, trustworthy pharmacist didn't]. To his credit, he ended the jab session with a thank you for the new information. No professional ego problem existed for this man. I'm lucky that I keep running into such health professionals. Just in case that's not happening for you right now, I thank The National Kidney Foundation for the following article.

Flu Season and Your Kidneys
By Leslie Spry, MD FACP FASN

As flu season approaches, kidney patients need to know what they can do and what they should avoid if they become ill. The first and most important action to take is to get a flu shot. All patients with Chronic Kidney Disease, including those with a kidney transplant should have a flu shot. Transplant patients may not have the nasal mist flu vaccine known as FluMist®. Transplant patients should have the regular injection for their flu vaccine. If you are a new transplant recipient, within the first 6 months, it is advisable to check with your transplant coordinator to make sure your transplant team allows flu shots in the first 6 months after transplant. ALL other kidney patients should receive a flu vaccination.

If the influenza virus is spreading in your community, there are medications that you can take to protect against influenza if you have not been vaccinated, however the dose of these medications may have to be modified for your level of kidney function. This is also true of antibiotics or any medication that you take for colds, bacterial infections or other viral infections. [I have written about this in **What Is It and How Did I Get It? Early Stage Chronic Kidney Disease** and the blog. You have to tell the prescribing physician about your CKD and/or remind him of it if (s)he already knows each time a prescription is written for you.] The doses of those medications may have to be modified for your level of kidney function. Even if you are vaccinated, it is still possible to get influenza and pneumonia, but the disease is usually much milder.

You should get plenty of rest and avoid other individuals who are ill, in order to limit the spread of the disease. If you are ill, stay home and rest.

You should drink plenty of fluids [Remember your limit on fluid intake] to stay well hydrated.

You should eat a balanced diet.

If you have gastrointestinal illness including nausea, vomiting or diarrhea, you should contact your physician. Immodium® is generally safe to take to control diarrhea. If you become constipated, medications that contain polyethylene glycol, such as Miralax® and Glycolax® are safe to take. You should avoid laxatives that contain magnesium and phosphates. Gastrointestinal illness can lead to dehydration or may keep you from taking your proper medication. If you are on a diuretic, it may not be a good idea to keep taking that diuretic if you are unable to keep liquids down or if you are experiencing diarrhea.

You should monitor you temperature and blood pressure carefully and report concerns to your physician.

Any medication you take should be reported to your physician.

Medications to avoid include all non-steroidal medications includ-ing ibuprofen, Motrin®, Advil®, Aleve®, and naproxen. Acetamino-phen (Tylenol® and others) and aspirin are generally safe to take with kidney disease. Acetaminophen doses should not ex-ceed 4000 milligrams per day [Nobody ever told me that! Why?]

If you take any of the over-the-counter medications, you should always drink plenty of water and stay well hydrated. If you take anti-histamines or decongestants, you should avoid those that contain ephedrine or pseudoephedrine.

Over-the-counter cold remedies that are safe to take for patients with high blood pressure are generally designated "HBP". Any over-the-counter medication that you take for a cold or flu should be approved by your doctor.

[There are more and different guidelines for those on dialysis, which I haven't included here.]

Dr. Rich Synder, DO – Guest Blog

11/21/11   I keep my eye out for any Chronic Kidney Disease pub-lications after the release date of my own book. One day, to my surprise since it had been a futile attempt until then, I dis-covered **_What You Must Know about Kidney Disease_**. I figured it was going to be about another kind of kidney disease just like all the others I'd looked at since last May, but it wasn't.

I bought it, read it, and as is my wont, contacted the author to both congratulate him on an informative book and ask him what-ever questions I had. It turned out Dr. Synder reads the blog and to quote him, "Concerning your blog, I love your blog!" Where's that feather that keeps knocking me over?

Below are the answers to some of the questions I asked him about probiotic and alkalinized water among other topics:

Let me clarify: **_Probiotics and alkalinized water are for everyone_**.

My approach: I am looking at the kidney as part of and working with your total body. It is a different approach than the way I was taught in fellowship. If the heart and the blood vessels and the cells are not working well, your kidneys are not going to work well. I am using a more holistic approach.

Probiotics in general: While decreasing total body inflammation, they help to normalize the immune system as well as help bowel irregularity. The kidney based probiotic is still a probiotic; it just also helps to also clear the intestine of the uremic toxins that can build up in advanced CKD. They have the lactobacillus and bifidobacterium species present in other probiotics.

Concerning water: Do you know how many people I see with early stage CKD who have a benign urine and no proteinuria? Why do they have early CKD? Maybe part of it is what we ingest and what we are exposed to every day. An article in *The New England Journal of Medicine* talked about water and low level lead exposure and how it can be a cause of CKD over the years. This encompasses the pesticides in the water, not to mention the cellular effect of an acidic Western diet. I did a show entitled "Are Colas Killing Your Kidneys?" in which I talked about the fact that twenty years of phosphoric acid are likely to have an effect on your kidneys.

Ongoing studies of how to treat glomerular disease and proteinuria: These look at protocols: what can I give – steroids or chemo or both? I am not going to say I have not used them or medications when necessary. I would be a hypocrite if I did. But....why, why, why do my patients have kidney disease and what can one do about it? The prevention is what we do each and every day of our lives.

Here are some suggestions:

1) ***Alkaline/anti-inflammatory based diet***: Some say, "Eat for your blood type." But, what is the DASH diet for hypertension? It is not just a low salt diet. It is also full of anti-oxidants and anti-inflammatory.

2) ***Water***: I have taken alkaline water myself and I notice a difference in how I feel. Our bodies are sixty percent water. Why would I not want to put the best type of water into it? Mineralized water helps with bone health. In alkalinized water, the hydroxyl ions produced from the reaction of the bicarbonate and the gastric acid with a low pH produce more hydroxyl ions which help buffer the acidity we produce on a daily basis. Where are these buffers? In the bones and in the cells, as well as some extracellular buffers. You are helping lower the total body acidity and decreasing the inflammation brought on by it. You do this early on so that you don't have a problem with advanced acidosis later. Why wait until you are acidotic before doing something?

3) ***Decreasing total body inflammation and raising anti-oxidant support***: Why is the heart the most common organ affected by kidney disease and dialysis? It's due to inflammation and vascular calcification. If a person is diabetic and obese, they may also have a fatty liver. Altered liver hemodynamics are also going to play a role in kidney function. I see the end aspect of this every day in the hospital. I look at these things too.

4) ***Standard care for someone with diabetes and kidney disease:*** This is the use of an ACE inhibitor. This is right and I use it with anyone I can. What happens if the person is on the ACE inhibitor and is still spilling tons of protein? What happens if they can't take the ACE inhibitor because of high potassium problems? I look for other answers.

Your kidney doctors are not wrong at all in what they are telling you. I just look at things from an additional perspective. Do I bat 1,000? No way. Have I had better results than before? Absolutely, yes. Do I need to learn a lot more? Heck, yes....I keep looking at things from a different perspective and asking why.

Psst! Want Some Herb?

11/28/11   When I was in college, all I heard between classes was, "Psst! Want some herb?" I thought I went to school for an education, but not exactly that kind. Since I was one of those kids who didn't know much about the world and wasn't ready to experiment, I stayed away from herb. Now I'm in my 60s and find I still need to stay away from herb – only the ingesting, not the smoking, kind. Intrigued? Read on.

Use of Herbal Supplements in Chronic Kidney Disease

As a Chronic Kidney Disease (CKD) patient, you may have considered the use of herbal products to assist you with various health concerns. This fact sheet will give you some information to enable you to make decisions regarding your use of herbs.

Use of herbal supplements may be unsafe for CKD patients, since your body is not able to clear waste products like a healthy person. There are some facts about herbs that every CKD patient should know:

- Very few herbs have been studied in CKD patients. What may be safe for healthy persons may not be safe for someone with CKD, and in fact, could be dangerous. Therefore, you need to be very cautious about your use of these products.
- The government does not regulate herbal supplements, so the exact content of these products is unknown.
- Without regulation, there are no requirements for testing, so the purity, safety and effectiveness of the products are unknown.
- Herbal preparations are subject to contamination (may contain toxic heavy metals such as lead or mercury).
- Products may contain minerals harmful to CKD patients, for example: potassium.

Some herbs that may serve as diuretics may also cause "kidney irritation" or damage. These include bucha leaves and juniper berries. Uva Ursi and parsley capsules may have negative side effects as well.

Many herbs can interact with prescription drugs. A few examples are St.Johns Wort, echinacea, ginkgo, garlic, ginseng, ginger, and blue cohosh. Transplant patients are especially at risk, as any interaction between herbs and medications could potentially put them at risk for rejection or losing the kidney. It is important to ask your doctor and/or pharmacist about any herbs or medicines you want to take to avoid potential problems.

Herbs that may be toxic to the kidneys

Artemisia absinthium (wormwood plant)	Periwinkle
Autumn crocus	Sassafras
Chuifong tuokuwan (Black Pearl)	Tung shueh
Horse chestnut	Vandelia cordifolia

Herbs that may be harmful in Chronic Kidney Disease

Alfalfa	Buckthorn	Ginger	Nettle
Aloe	Capsicum	Ginseng	Noni juice
Bayberry	Cascara	Horsetail	Panax
Blue Cohosh	Coltsfoot	Licorice	Rhubarb
Broom	Dandelion	Mate	Senna
			Vervain

Herbs known to be unsafe for all people

Chapparal	Pennyroyal
Comfrey	Pokeroot
Ephedra (Ma Huang)	Sassafras
Lobelia	Senna
Mandrake	Yohimbe

These lists are not necessarily complete. More information regarding the use of herbs will become available over time. You are encouraged to proceed with caution with *all* herbal preparations and use them only under the direction of your medical team.

With all of these cautions, perhaps you are wondering if use of any herbs is a good idea. The use of common herbs, in normal amounts, when cooking is just fine and typically recommended to enhance the flavor of foods on a low-sodium diet.

So, before you take any herbal supplement, we recommend:
- Checking with your doctor, dietitian, pharmacist and/or product manufacturer regarding safety, dosage, duration of use, interactions with prescription drugs, etc.
- Use only standardized herbal extracts made by reputable companies.
- **Never** take more than the recommended dosage, or longer than recommended.
- Do not use herbal remedies for serious illness.
- Do not use herbs if considering pregnancy.

Remember ... natural does not mean safe, especially for CKD patients. Be smart and ask questions before using any herbal products.

The following references can provide additional information regarding the use of herbal supplements.

Online:
American Botanical Council

National Center for Complementary and Alternative Medicine

National Library of Medicine, Medline Plus

United States Pharmacopeial

In print:
PDR for Herbal Medicines. Gruenwald J, Bendler T, Jaenicke C, eds. Montvale NJ: Medical Economics Company, Inc., 2000

The Honest Herbal. Tyler V. Pharmaceutical Products Press, New York, 1999

[I've noticed Senna in quite a few weight loss and appetite reduction products. Stay away from those.]

Pollyanna Lives... In An Artificial Kidney

12/5/11 It's amazing how long a week can be sometimes. This week felt longer because I was not careful about overdoing, over-did, and spent two days in bed [Well, that part of it was great: DVDs, books, phone conversations, a little internet]. I've learned my lesson... I think.

I have this vague recollection of saying the same thing July 4th weekend when we went up to Prescott for the rodeo and parade but ended up in the hotel room pandering to my negligent energy level instead. Okay, maybe this time I really have learned my lesson – at least, until next time. Some lessons are hard to learn, but I'm hopeful. Hmmm, have I mentioned my kids refer to me as Pollyanna?

Talking about Pollyanna, I found this article in *Renal & Urology News* and started hopping up and down with excitement – while trying to stay seated at the computer. I'm not exactly a kid and am distressed at the thought of having my children disrupt their lives – if they're even matches – when and if I need a kidney. My brothers and my fiancé are all older than I am and, logically although sadly, might not be around at that time. So who will donate their live kidney to me should the need arise? If not a living donor, won't I be placed on the list to wait... and wait... and wait? Maybe not. Here's hope.

Nephrologists and Urologists Collaborate on Implantable Artificial Kidney

Kenneth W. Angermeier, MD, James Simon, MD, Hadley M. Wood, MD

Four years ago, a joint effort was established between nephrologists and urologists at the Cleveland Clinic Glickman Urological and Kidney Institute to develop and implant a bioartificial kidney. The bioartificial kidney uses a high-efficiency biomimetic silicon nanopore filter that acts synonymously as a glomerulus, in combination with a kidney epithelial cell bioreactor that allows for reabsorption of essential electrolytes from plasma filtrate.... A Phase 2 trial of an extracorporeal system utilizing these technologies was completed in 2005. Current efforts have been aimed at miniaturization of technology to facilitate implantation of a miniaturized biohybrid device.

This project has been funded by the National Institute of Biomedical Imaging and Bioengineering, the Wildwood Foundation, Cleveland Clinic, and the University of California, San Francisco. Nephrologists and engineers involved with inception and initial development of the project include William H. Fissell, MD (Cleveland Clinic), Aaron J. Fleischman, PhD, (Cleveland Clinic), Shuvo Roy, PhD (University of California, San Francisco) and H. David Humes, MD (University of Michigan). At Cleveland Clinic, Dr. Fissell, a clinical nephrologist, has teamed with Matthew N. Simmons, MD, PhD, a urologic oncologist to develop prototypes suitable for surgical implantation. Dr Fissell has a background in biomedical engineering and oversees design and construction of the components of the device. Together, Drs. Fissell and Simmons work through the processes of design modification, surgical implantation, *in vivo* device maintenance, and functional monitoring. To date they have implanted four hemofilter devices, the last of which remained *in vivo* for five days.

This project is a model example of the advantages of direct partnership between nephrology and urology colleagues. Dr. Fissell and colleagues provide expertise in terms of materials engineering and renal physiology to develop a device capable of reproducing kidney function. In partnership with Dr. Simmons and the urology team, they are steadily advancing the transformation of the device from concept to an implantable reality. It is hoped that the success of this research may eventually impact the lives of millions of patients with kidney disease.

Will This Really Be Possible?

12/12/11   Are you so busy in this period between Thanksgiving and Chanukah/ Christmas/Kwanzaa/whatever other celebration I don't know about that you haven't had the chance to keep up with the Chronic Kidney Disease world? Relax: that's what this blog is for. Besides, this may very well be a gift for you – albeit not this year. Honestly, I'd settle for this gift any time before I hit the need for dialysis.

If you've read ***What Is It and How Did I Get It? Early Stage Chronic Kidney Disease*** or the earliest ***SlowItDownCKD*** blogs, you know I have an irrational revulsion toward dialysis. It's an emotional reaction and one that rears its ugly head every time I think about the process.

Maybe I don't have to have that reaction any more. Maybe dialysis won't be necessary any more. I know I sound delusional, but let's hold off on that opinion until after you read this article from MedIndia. It's a bit long, but well worth the read.

Hope for Treating Chronic Kidney Disease Via Regeneration of Specialized Cells

Podocytes are specialized type of epithelial cells in the kidney, which get damaged in more than 90 percent of all Chronic Kidney Disease cases. Now researchers at the Stanford University School of Medicine have uncovered an unexpected pathway that reveals for the first time how these cells may regenerate and renew themselves during normal kidney function.

This finding is an important step toward one day therapeutically coaxing the cells to divide, which could be used to treat people with Chronic Kidney Disease.

"Researchers have studied these cells for years, but the prevailing view has been that they don't renew themselves," said associate professor of medicine Steven Artandi, MD, PhD. "Now we've found that podocytes can enter and leave the cell cycle in response to certain common signaling pathways."

Artandi is the senior author of the study, which will be published online Dec. 4 in Nature Medicine. The first author of the work is former post-doctoral scholar Marina Shkreli, PhD, who is now at the Laboratory of Biology and Pathology of Genomes at the University of Nice in France.

Podocytes are found only in the kidney and are an integral structural component of its blood-filtering system. They stand shoulder-to-shoulder in a part of the organ called the glomerulus and wrap their long "feet" around the semi-permeable capillaries through which blood flows. Narrow slits between the feet allow small molecules, such as water and salts, to pass while blocking large proteins.

This filtering process is the first step to forming urine, and it is critically important — even one missing cell can leave a gap that would allow unwanted molecules through the barrier. (Imagine wrapping your hands around a length of leaky garden hose so that the water seeps out between your fingers. Lift up one finger and you're liable to get sprayed in the face.)

This may be why previous researchers searching for signs of self-renewal in podocytes were unsuccessful, because any such renewal or replacement would likely need to be carefully orchestrated to avoid compromising the filtration system. As a result, scientists have been forced to conclude that the podocytes rarely, if ever, divided.

"It used to be thought that you were born with podocytes, and you died with the same podocytes — you don't make any more during your lifetime," said Artandi. The only exception was certain rare types of kidney disease in which the podocytes abandon their blood-filtration duties en masse to de-differentiate into less-specialized, dividing cells that little resemble their predecessors. As a result, the glomerulus collapses and the patients' kidneys begin to fail. One such disease is HIV-associated nephropathy, or HIVAN.

The problem was, such a scenario doesn't make a lot of evolutionary sense — particularly when other epithelial cells routinely regenerate themselves. "Podocytes are vitally important, and are also under enormous physical stress," said Artandi. "It's hard to understand why we would have such a vulnerable blood-filtration system."

To understand more about kidney biology, Artandi and Shkreli investigated the role of a protein component of the telomerase complex called TERT. Although telomerase is best known as an enzyme involved in cell aging, recent research in Artandi's lab and others have shown that TERT also plays a role in many types of cellular regeneration. The researchers found that temporarily increasing the expression of TERT in adult, otherwise healthy laboratory mice caused the formerly stolid podocytes to abruptly de-differentiate and begin dividing. As a result, the glomerulus collapsed in a way that resembles what happens in humans with HIVAN. Conversely, ceasing the overexpression allowed the cells to stop dividing, re-specialize and resume their normal functions.

When Artandi and Shkreli looked closely at the glomeruli in humans with HIVAN, they found that TERT expression was increased. Equally important, the Wnt signaling pathway, which is important in embryonic development and in the self-renewal of stem cells, was also activated (Previous research in the Artandi lab has linked telomerase activity to the Wnt pathway.) blocking Wnt signaling in a mouse model of HIVAN also stopped the podocytes from dividing and improved their function. "The implication is that podocytes may utilize recognized pathways of regeneration to renew themselves throughout life," said Artandi. People suffering from Chronic Kidney Disease may simply have worn out or outpaced their podocytes' capacity for renewal, he believes.

Now that the researchers know podocytes have the ability [to] regenerate in response to common cellular signals, their next step is to learn whether this regeneration occurs in healthy animals and people. "If we can harness this regeneration," Artandi said, "we may one day be able to treat people with Chronic Kidney Disease."

How Sweet It Is... Or Is It?

12/19/11 Thanksgiving is over and I thought I'd learn from that not so successful experience [as far as energy and proper eating only – it was a delicious experience having my step-daughter to ourselves], but I'm not so sure I have. Hence, excerpts from two helpful articles.

When I scan the internet for articles to present on the blog, I usually end up finding some that help me with my own difficult areas. Odd how the universe takes care of you, isn't it? I raised my children to believe that things happen for a reason whether we know the reason or not, and am so gratified to hear them remind me of that time after time. You'll understand as you read today's blog.

This first bit is from foodconsumer.org.

Fructose Raises Risk for Kidney Disease, Hypertension
Eating too much fructose may cause a series of diseases including fatty liver, insulin resistance or diabetes, dyslipidemia, hypertension and kidney disease, according to a report in the Nov 2011 issue of *International Journal of Nephrology*. In the report, Marek Kretowicz of Nicolaus Copernicus University in Torun Poland and colleagues reviewed 62 studies and concluded that studies suggest that excessive fructose intake may be one of the causes for the current epidemic of obesity, diabetes and cardiorenal disease. Fructose is a monosaccharide present in sucrose (beet sugar, cane sugar etc.), high fructose corn syrup (hfcs), honey and fruits.

The researchers cited studies as suggesting that not all fructose sources are the same. Not all sources of fructose cause diabetes, kidney disease and cardiovascular disease. The researchers said natural sources of fructose such as fruits are rich in beneficial nutrients like antioxidants, vitamin C or ascorbic acid, polyphenols, potassium, and fiber that may counter the adverse effect of fructose. Previous studies found fructose intake was not correlated with increased risk of high blood pressure or hypertension in a population in which much of the fructose intake came from fruits. However, the association was found significant when the fructose from fruits was excluded. According to the report, fructose can cause fatty liver and glycogen accumulation, insulin resistance and islet dysfunction, obesity, hypertension and vascular disease, and kidney disease.

Get the message? Fruit, not candy or cakes. Now where have I heard that before? I know a great deal of my problem with cele-brations is that, not only do others not understand that I don't have the energy I used to [Say, isn't that true of a great many people who are not ill, simply aging?], but half the time I don't, so the day of the dinner, party, etc. comes and I'm too tired from the preparations to enjoy it. I've got to grow up and stop this ri-diculous cycle.

Then there's this except from KevinMD.

Living with chronic illness during the holiday season
....Bottom line, suffering from a chronic condition can be an ongoing crisis—for you and for those you're close to. That crisis can come to a head during the holidays when people's expecta-tions of one another are high and when stress levels for everyone are likely to be off the charts for any number of reasons—health, financial, relationship issues. ....when the holidays arrive, you're suddenly thrust into the middle of a lively and chaotic social scene where you're expected to participate in a range of activities, often for days in a row.

A bit of advance warning to loved-ones can go a long way toward minimizing stress levels over unrealistic expectations....If you're one of the many people with chronic health problems who don't *look* sick, the initiative is with you to *make your condition visible*. Here are some suggestions for helping loved-ones understand what your life is like and for giving them a heads-up on what to expect from you during the holidays.

Share information with them from the Internet or from books
Often the best way to educate loved-ones about chronic pain and illness is to use a neutral source because it takes the emotional impact out of the communication….. Print out select pages or forward a few links to family and close friends. Alternatively, if you have a book about your condition [Like ***What Is It and How Did I Get It? Early Stage Chronic Kidney Disease***], photo-copy the pages that cover what you'd like them to know about you. In your accompanying note, keep it "light"—you could joke that "there won't be a test." But also make it clear that this favor you're asking is important to you.

Write a letter
….Without complaining, express how difficult it's been for you to adjust to this unexpected change in your life and how you wish you could be as active as you once were during the holidays….I would end by telling them what to expect from you during the holidays—that you may have to skip some events, that you may have to excuse yourself right after eating to go lie down, that you may have to come late and leave early. In my experience, spelling out my limitations ahead of time is helpful not just to others, but to me, because I find it much easier to exercise the self-discipline it takes to excuse myself from a room full of people if I know that at least some of them are already expecting it….

Find that ONE ally and enlist his or her help
….It's so helpful for me to be "prompted" by my ally because, when I start to overdo things, adrenaline kicks in which fools me into thinking I'm doing fine. But using adrenaline to get by just sets me up for a bad crash later on. Your ally may be a close friend or family member who's just waiting for you to enlist his or her help. Think long and hard before you decide there's no such person in your life.

In the end, you may have to recognize that some loved-ones may never accept your limitations
….Just as you can't force people to love you, you can't force people to accept you. But getting angry at them just exacerbates your own symptoms. That's why it's important to protect yourself from allowing their lack of understanding to continually upset you.
Think of it as protecting yourself from another chronic condition: chronic anger….

Thank you to both contributing authors for helping me understand my life at this time of the year.

Po...Pot...Potassium? What's that?

12/26/11 While celebrating the season with dinners in restaurants, I heard this question several times: "What's with you and potassium?" Just as I was framing an original post on this very subject, The National Kidney Foundation posted their potassium fact sheet. Nothing like learning from the masters.

What is potassium and why is it important to you?
Potassium is a mineral found in many of the foods you eat. It plays a role in keeping your heartbeat regular and your muscles working right. It is the job of healthy kidneys to keep the right amount of potassium in your body. However, when your kidneys are not healthy, you often need to limit certain foods that can increase the potassium in your blood to a dangerous level. You may feel some weakness, numbness and tingling if your potassium is at a high level. **If your potassium becomes too high, it can cause an irregular heartbeat or a heart attack.**

What is a safe level of potassium in my blood?
Ask your doctor or dietitian about your monthly blood potassium level and enter it here:

If it is 3.5-5.0…………………………….You are in the **SAFE** zone
If it is 5.1-6.0………………………………You are in the **CAUTION** zone
If it is higher than 6.0………………You are in the **DANGER** zone

How can I keep my potassium level from getting too high?
- You should limit foods that are high in potassium. Your renal dietitian will help you plan your diet so you are getting the right amount of potassium.
- Eat a variety of foods but in moderation.
- If you want to include some high potassium vegetables in your diet, leach them before using. Leaching is a process by which some potassium can be pulled out of the vegetable.

Instructions for leaching selected high potassium vegetables can be found at the end of this fact sheet. Check with your dietitian on the amount of leached high potassium vegetables that can be safely included in your diet.

- Do not drink or use the liquid from canned vegetables, or the juices from cooked meat.
- Remember that almost all foods have some potassium. The size of the serving is very important. A large amount of a low potassium food can turn into a high-potassium food.
- If you are on dialysis, be sure to get all the treatment or exchanges prescribed to you.

(There are so many high potassium and low potassium food lists online these days, as well as telephone apps that will count food potassium levels, that I've omitted such lists from this blog.)

How do I get some of the potassium out of my favorite high-potassium vegetables?

The process of leaching will help pull potassium out of some high-potassium vegetables. It is important to remember that leaching will not pull all of the potassium out of the vegetable. You must still limit the amount of leached high-potassium vegetables you eat. Ask your dietitian about the amount of leached vegetables that you can safely have in your diet.

How to leach vegetables.

For Potatoes, Sweet Potatoes, Carrots, Beets, and Rutabagas:

1. Peel and place the vegetable in cold water so they won't darken.
2. Slice vegetable 1/8 inch thick.
3. Rinse in warm water for a few seconds.
4. Soak for a minimum of two hours in warm water. Use ten times the amount of water to the amount of vegetables. If soaking longer, change the water every four hours.
5. Rinse under warm water again for a few seconds.

6. Cook vegetable with five times the amount of water to the amount of vegetable.

For Squash, Mushrooms, Cauliflower, and Frozen Greens:
1. Allow frozen vegetable to thaw to room temperature and drain.
2. Rinse fresh or frozen vegetables in warm water for a few seconds.
3. Soak for a minimum of two hours in warm water. Use ten times the amount of water to the amount of vegetables. If soaking longer, change the water every four hours.
4. Rinse under warm water again for a few seconds.
5. Cook the usual way, but with five times the amount of water to the amount of vegetable.

Until next year,
Keep living your life!

Index

A

B

C

D

E

F

G

H

T

Technology, 113-5
Testing, 30, 50-1
Toxins, 48-9, 167
Transplant, 31-8, 65, 108,
    164, 171
Twenty Four Hour Urine Col-
lection, 50-6

V

Vegetables and Fruits, See
    Fruits and Vegetables

Vegetarian, 59-61
Vytorin, 71-3

W

Waistline, 121-3
Water, 48-9, 79-81, 143-4
    (Also see Alkalinized Wa-
    ter)
World Kidney Day, 16-7, 24

Z

Zebra Fish, 41-2

Additional reviews for *What Is It and How Did I Get It? Early Stage Chronic Kidney Disease*

"I've had this book in paperback for a while and when Amazon offered me the option to buy the digital version at a discounted price since I had purchased the paperback from them, I jumped at it. I'm a sucker for loaning out hard copy and this way if I find a fellow kidney disease sufferer, I can let them have my paperback and I will always have my digital backup for reference. This is a great book by a fellow kidney disease patient who also publishes a very good blog. There are so many details to track with this disease and she talks about the daily life of it. Very helpful and answers so many questions. She's a born researcher, so all her information has backup links to let you know this is authentic medical advice to get some of those questions answered between doctor's visits."

"Gail Rae has provided a good insight to the bombshell that befalls millions of unsuspecting humans worldwide. A CKD victim myself with years of experience under my belt, found the book extremely informative and a great reference when providing peer support to newly diagnosed sufferers of this silent killer."

"I was just diagnosed with Chronic Kidney disease Stage 4 a few weeks ago and I want to THANK YOU very much for this book. I put it on my Kindle. It is written in a way that one newly diagnosed and not in the medical field can understand."

"Ms. Rae knows, in my opinion, what she is talking about. She is direct-to the point-and the book is easily understood. She has just a hint of humor in her writing which keeps the reader engaged. Will keep this in my reference library."

"It is written for a patient like us, mean that the language it is simple and easy to understand, good sense of humor and a positive aptitude with this silent killer, another book that deserve a place on your personal library. Very informative, excellent book."

"Great book to help with the anxiety that comes with the diagnosis"

"So much good information for Chronic Kidney Disease Patients, from beginning to end. Thank you Gail Rae."

"One of the best on the subject not so much for the info but the way it was presented. Almost like a novel. Makes you forget your kidney is not behaving the way it should."

"A book that is very helpful to CKD3 patients. It gives the facts and figures needed most to those with this condition!"

"Very helpful"

"This is not a medical book, but it is the ONLY book I could find discussing the issue of early stage CKD. My twenty month old son was diagnosed on Thursday, almost in passing by his nephrologist. I did not ask any questions on CKD, I was not handed any pamphlets - I went into shock and reacted like I always do to bad news I cannot process. I asked questions about my infant son's high blood pressure (the reason for the appointment). Tried to pay attention, remained calm so as not to upset my children who were with us in the room, and then began to research like crazy. I also went back to the doctor and confirmed that she had in fact diagnosed my son with CKD (stage 1). So for me this book has been very helpful, but again I am still in a shock like state and just want to know how to slow the progression of the disease so that my son can have a mostly normal childhood. Best I can tell there is no treatment for the early stages and at least my son's nephrologist (who is an expert in the area) does not appear to be at all concerned or worried. So I appreciate this book because it reminded me to take the reins (no one else will or can) and I plan to speak to my son's pharmacist today about his other daily prescriptions, just to make sure that it's okay to take... I plan to get more knowl-edgeable about nutrition (just like the author did) but most of all I plan to let my son play the sports he loves because activity is so important (the author loves to dance, my son loves to try and ice skate like his big sister).

This book is a very quick read, it's almost like you are having a conversation with a friend over coffee. It calmed me down, it gave me direction and it was available on my kindle in seconds. THANK YOU!!!!"

My Notes -

Have you read my other Chronic Kidney Disease books?
available on Amazon.com and B&N.com
(print and digital)

What Is It and How Did I Get It?
Early Stage Chronic Kidney Disease
SlowItDownCKD 2012
SlowItDownCKD 2013
SlowItDownCKD 2014
SlowItDownCKD 2015
SlowItDownCKD 2016

Follow the blog at
https://gailraegarwood.wordpress.com

SLOWITDOWNCKD
EARLY AND MODERATE STAGE CHRONIC KIDNEY DISEASE

On Instagram, Pinterest, and Twitter go to
@SlowItDownCKD

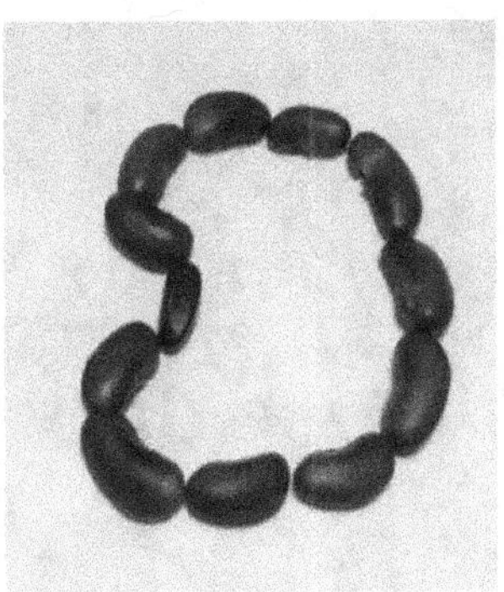

And then, there's the Facebook page at
https://www.facebook.com/SlowItDownCKD/

Don't forget you can email me at
SlowItDownCKD@gmail.com

If you'd like to read a time travel romance
(available on Amazon.com
in both digital and print)

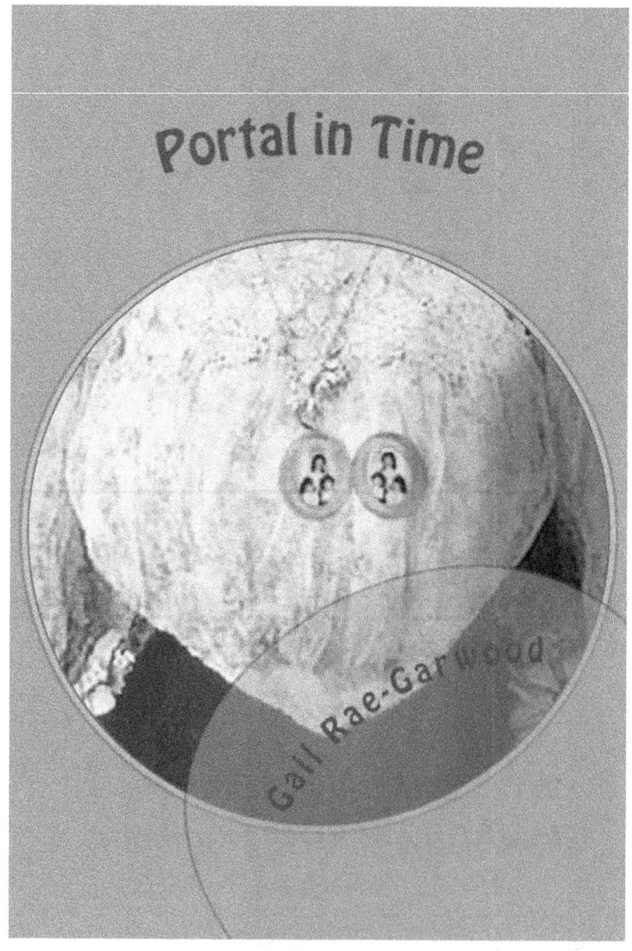